T0252730

Susan Taylor-Brown, PhD, M[...]
Alejandro Garcia, PhD
Editors

HIV Affected
and Vulnerable Youth:
Prevention Issues
and Approaches

HIV Affected and Vulnerable Youth: Prevention Issues and Approaches has been co-published simultaneously as *Journal of HIV/AIDS Prevention & Education for Adolescents & Children*, Volume 3, Numbers 1/2 1999.

Pre-publication
REVIEWS,
COMMENTARIES,
EVALUATIONS . . .

"**T**his compilation of research is long overdue for a nearly forgotten population. Human service workers and social workers will benefit from the illuminating outcomes which will influence future' social work interventions."

Evelyn R. Blackburn, MSW, CSW, ACSW
Director of Community Services
Community Health Network
Rochester, NY

"**I** found that the book dealt with the issues regarding AIDS/HIV, women, children and adolescents in a concise, positive and informative manner. There are sections that go into detail on the various issues facing women who are not only single parents, most often minority and marginalized already but also dealing with stigma of HIV disease. The studies and findings written about confirm the courage I have seen with the HIV positive women I work with in dealing with their illness. The articles also address the multitude of issues facing the children in these families. There is a wealth of information that I will be able to use as I put together presentations on women/families as well as in my role of helping families incorporate permanency planning into their lives.

The sections on adolescents, infected or affected by AIDS/HIV accessing services presents an accurate account of the challenges adolescents face in the age of AIDS. Having worked with many adolescents, I know how important it is that they be able to access services in a non-threatening, non-judgemental environment. Not only are they facing their own vulnerability to the disease, but they must face the probability of losing a parent and/or becoming caregivers to either parents or siblings. Professionals working with HIV positive women with children and/or adolescents will find the materials in the book informative and useful as they help families especially children and adolescents, deal with the impact of HIV and what it means to the family."

Jane D. Hallinen, BS
AIDS Services Director
Catholic Charities Community
Residential Services
Diocese of Rochester, NY

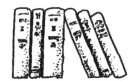

More pre-publication
REVIEWS, COMMENTARIES, EVALUATIONS . . .

"**T**his distinguished panel of authors has produced a scholarly work of high quality with thoughtful attention to the social and psychological issues that face young people. The guidelines for practice challenge the reader to consider the varied and complex issues that young people face in general and in the wake of the dis-ease of HIV. Cultural issues, both in terms of race and ethnicity as well as the "culture of adolescence" and the "culture of the affected," are woven throughout the book in natural and unique ways.

The work is innovative. The editors, in their selection of topics to be addressed as well as the researchers/practitioners who author the chapters, stimulate and challenge the reader to think critically about the issues for vulnerable youth and their families. Their findings and recommendations cannot help but bring us to the point of looking around and within ourselves for paradigm shifts that will bring about creative changes in the ways we think about and work with youth and in their behalf.

The work is easily read and the content is appealing to varied audiences, from researcher to policy maker, from practitioner to grass-roots advocate. It is refreshing to see a work that so nicely bridges research, policy and practice in reader-friendly format and style. Bold and daring in its illumination of the scope and depth of the issues for youth and their families, presented in ways that are stark, yet hopeful, this book is an excellent reference for any one who works with and cares about our youth."

Patricia A. Stewart, MSS ASCW, LSW
Assistant Professor
Department of Sociology
Social Work and Criminal Justice
La Salle University
Philadelphia, PA

More pre-publication
REVIEWS, COMMENTARIES, EVALUATIONS . . .

"This book represents a major contribution to the literature in the area of HIV affected and vulnerable youth. Chapters of the book report on significant research recently conducted in this area and further our understanding of youth and HIV disease. Of special interest is the recurring finding of great resiliency on the part of affected youth and their families, something which should be of interest to direct service providers and program planners alike.

The research which is reported here is well constructed, with a combination of large and small sample studies. In addition, quantitative as well as qualitative methods are utilized. This is a sophisticated volume which should appeal to academic as well as to direct practice audiences."

Vincent J. Lynch, DSW
Director
National Research & Training Center
On Social Work and HIV/AIDS
Boston College
Chestnut Hill, MA

"The different perspectives represented in this book contribute in a refreshing way to our understanding of how HIV/AIDS is impacting children/youth and their families. Empirical and descriptive studies provide applied knowledge about the needs and resiliency of children/youth from diverse backgrounds and environments. This book is a must for child welfare practitioners, HIV/AIDS researchers, academicians teaching courses about children and youth courses, and pubic health workers."

Flavio F. Marsiglia
Assistant Professor
School of Social Work
Arizona State University

More pre-publication
REVIEWS, COMMENTARIES, EVALUATIONS . . .

"While reading *HIV Affected and Vulnerable Youth: Prevention Issues and Approaches*, all I could think about is that this is about time. Adolescents and youth are one of those disenfranchised groups that have no voice or lack the power to make their needs heard. All health professionals dealing with youth might want to question what they can do to help prevent HIV; this book helps being that into the light. All youth are clearly at risk. Discussing sex and sexuality does not mean endorsing sexual activity, but the continued lack of discussion only increases the risks, increasing the spread of HIV. It will only help us in addressing our taboos, too, by breaking the silence among our adolescents."

Peter Lesko, MSW
Social Work Case-Manager
Library Resources
DePalmer House
Syracuse

HIV Affected
and Vulnerable Youth:
Prevention Issues
and Approaches

HIV Affected and Vulnerable Youth: Prevention Issues and Approaches has been co-published simultaneously as *Journal of HIV/AIDS Prevention & Education for Adolescents & Children,* Volume 3, Numbers 1/2 1999.

HIV Affected and Vulnerable Youth: Prevention Issues and Approaches

Susan Taylor-Brown, PhD, MPH, ACSW
Alejandro Garcia, PhD
Editors

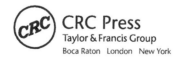

CRC Press
Taylor & Francis Group
Boca Raton   London   New York

CRC Press is an imprint of the
Taylor & Francis Group, an informa business

Reprinted 2010 by CRC Press
CRC Press
6000 Broken Sound Parkway, NW
Suite 300, Boca Raton, FL 33487
270 Madison Avenue
New York, NY 10016
2 Park Square, Milton Park
Abingdon, Oxon OX14 4RN, UK

HIV Affected and Vulnerable Youth: Prevention Issues and Approaches has been co-published simultaneously as *Journal of HIV/AIDS Prevention & Education for Adolescents & Children,* Volume 3, Numbers 1/2 1999.

© 1999 by The Haworth Press, Inc. All rights reserved. No part of this work may be reproduced or utilized in any form or by any means, electronic or mechanical, including photocopying, microfilm and recording, or by any information storage and retrieval system, without permission in writing from the publisher. Printed in the United States of America. Reprint - 2007

The development, preparation, and publication of this work has been undertaken with great care. However, the publisher, employees, editors, and agents of The Haworth Press and all imprints of The Haworth Press, Inc., including The Haworth Medical Press® and The Pharmaceutical Products Press®, are not responsible for any errors contained herein or for consequences that may ensue from use of materials or information contained in this work. Opinions expressed by the author(s) are not necessarily those of The Haworth Press, Inc.

Cover design by Thomas J. Mayshock Jr.

Library of Congress Cataloging-in-Publication Data

HIV affected and vulnerable youth: prevention issues and approaches / Susan Taylor-Brown, Alejandro Garcia, editors.
    p. cm.
    "Co-published simultaneously as Journal of HIV/AIDS prevention & education for adolescents & children, volume 3, numbers 1/2 1999."
    Includes bibliographical references and index.
    ISBN 0-7890-0792-4 (alk. paper)–ISBN 0-7890-0825-4 (alk. paper)
    1. AIDS (Disease) in adolescence–Prevention. 2. HIV infections–Prevention. 3. Children of AIDS patients–Services for. I. Taylor-Brown, Susan. II. Garcia, Alejandro.
RJ387.A25.H567 1999
362.1′969792′00835–dc21
                                              99-046617

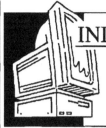

INDEXING & ABSTRACTING

Contributions to this publication are selectively indexed or abstracted in print, electronic, online, or CD-ROM version(s) of the reference tools and information services listed below. This list is current as of the copyright date of this publication. See the end of this section for additional notes.

- *AIDS Abstracts*
- *AIDS Info Docu Schweiz*
- *AIDS Reference Guide*
- *AIDS Targeted Information*
- *Applied Social Sciences Index & Abstracts (ASSIA) (Online: ASSI via Data-Star) (CD-Rom: ASSIA Plus)*
- *BUBL Information Service, an Internet-based Information Service for the UK higher education community*
- *Cambridge Scientific Abstracts*
- *CINAHL (Cumulative Index to Nursing & Allied Health Literature)*
- *CNPIEC Reference Guide: Chinese National Directory of Foreign Periodicals*
- *Current Medical Literature-Infectious Diseases*
- *EMBASE/Excerpta Medica/Secondary Publishing Division*
- *ERIC Clearinghouse on Teaching & Teacher Education*
- *Family Studies Database (online and CD/ROM)*
- *Guide to Social Science & Religion*
- *Health Management Information Service (HELMIS)*
- *HealthPromis*
- *HOMODOK/"Relevant" Bibliographic database, Documentation Centre for Gay & Lesbian Studies, University of Amsterdam (selective printed abstracts in "Homologie" and bibliographic computer databases covering cultural, historical, social and political aspects of gay & lesbian topics)*

(continued)

- *Leeds Medical Information*
- *Mental Health Abstracts (online through DIALOG)*
- *PASCAL, c/o Institute de L'Information Scientifique et Technique. Cross-disciplinary electronic database covering the fields of science, technology & medicine. Also available on CD-ROM, and can generate customized retrospective searches*
- *Referativnyi Zhurnal (Abstracts Journal of the All-Russian Institute of Scientific and Technical Information)*
- *Sage Family Studies Abstracts (SFSA)*
- *Studies on Women Abstracts*

Special Bibliographic Notes related to special journal issues (separates) and indexing/abstracting:

- indexing/abstracting services in this list will also cover material in any "separate" that is co-published simultaneously with Haworth's special thematic journal issue or DocuSerial. Indexing/abstracting usually covers material at the article/chapter level.
- monographic co-editions are intended for either non-subscribers or libraries which intend to purchase a second copy for their circulating collections.
- monographic co-editions are reported to all jobbers/wholesalers/approval plans. The source journal is listed as the "series" to assist the prevention of duplicate purchasing in the same manner utilized for books-in-series.
- to facilitate user/access services all indexing/abstracting services are encouraged to utilize the co-indexing entry note indicated at the bottom of the first page of each article/chapter/contribution.
- this is intended to assist a library user of any reference tool (whether print, electronic, online, or CD-ROM) to locate the monographic version if the library has purchased this version but not a subscription to the source journal.
- individual articles/chapters in any Haworth publication are also available through the Haworth Document Delivery Service (HDDS).

ABOUT THE EDITORS

Susan Taylor-Brown, PhD, MPH, ACSW, is Associate Professor in the School of Social Work at Syracuse University in Syracuse, New York. She is also Chair of the health care concentration at the University and teaches in the areas of human behavior and social environment, practice, and health. Since 1986, Dr. Taylor-Brown has been developing services for HIV-infected parents and their children and she consults with local and National AIDS services providers and is active in other HIV/AIDS-related activities. She is an associate of the National Center for HIV/AIDS Training and Research at Boston College; member of the Child Welfare League of America National Task Force on HIV Infection in Children, Adolescents and Families; member of the AIDS/HIV committee at the University; member of the planning committee for the Eleventh Annual HIV/AIDS: The Social Work Response Conference; and serves as the New York State AIDS liaison to the National Association of Social Workers. As a member of the National Coalition for the Education of Health Professionals in Genetics (NCHPEG), Dr. Taylor-Brown is advocating for social wok inclusion in the services provided to families considering genetic testing. Her areas of interest include HIV/AIDS research focusing on helping HIV-affected children cope with parental illness and permanency planning needs, how women are coping with the disease, the use of videotapes in preserving the family's history for surviving children, and the sources of satisfaction and strain for long-term HIV/AIDS workers.

Alejandro Garcia, PhD, is Professor in the School of Social Work at Syracuse University, where he chairs the gerontology concentration and teaches in the areas of social policy and human diversity. He currently serves as Chairman of the Board of Directors for the National Hispanic Council on Aging and as Secretary of the New York State Communities Aid Association (SCAA). Dr. Garcia presently serves on the editorial board of *The Journal of Sociology and Social Welfare* and is the book review editor of *The Journal of Multicultural Social Work.* He also serves as consulting editor of *The Journal of Social Work Education* and *Social Work, The Journal of the National Association of Social Workers.*

Dr. Garcia has been the recipient of a number of honors, the most recent being a scholarship named in his honor by the division of social work at the California State University at Sacramento. He was also recognized with the Distinguished Social Work Educator of the Decade Award from the social work division of the California State University at Sacramento in September 1997.

To my parents, Josefina L. Garcia and the late Arturo C. Garcia, for their love, guidance and support throughout my life.

Alejandro Garcia

To the many families who have shared their experiences living with HIV with me and to my family–David, Marian and Marc for their loving support.

Susan Taylor-Brown

HIV Affected and Vulnerable Youth: Prevention Issues and Approaches

CONTENTS

Foreword

Our work with families whose lives have been touched by HIV/ AIDS inspired us to develop a publication addressing the unique needs of HIV affected and vulnerable youth from heavily affected communities. HIV disease is having a profound effect upon our youth; yet, the impact of HIV disease on children and adolescents continues to receive less attention than deserved. As we approach the end of the second decade of the pandemic, we now have a generation of children who have only known a world in which HIV disease is part of the societal fabric. These children and adolescents are particularly vulnerable to becoming HIV infected themselves, and all are affected by the disease within their families and communities.

To live in a family in which a family member is HIV-infected means increased vulnerability for the children and youth in the family. Children and adolescents whose parents who are HIV+ are challenged to grow and develop in the face of uncertainty regarding their parents' and in turn, their own futures. Children in such homes find themselves faced with illness, disability, and the possibility of death of one or more family members. To lose a parent is recognized as a major developmental challenge. To lose both parents and/or other relatives is incomprehensible for most; yet, for far too many HIV affected children, this is their reality. In such homes, there is a higher

Susan Taylor-Brown, PhD, MPH, ACSW, is Associate Professor, School of Social Work, Syracuse University, Syracuse, NY.

Alejandro Garcia, PhD, is Professor, School of Social Work, Syracuse University, Syracuse, NY.

[Haworth co-indexing entry note]: "Foreword." Taylor-Brown, Susan, and Alejandro Garcia. Co-published simultaneously in *Journal of HIV/AIDS Prevention & Education for Adolescents & Children* (The Haworth Press, Inc.) Vol. 3, No. 1/2, 1999, pp. xv-xvii; and: *HIV Affected and Vulnerable Youth: Prevention Issues and Approaches* (ed: Susan Taylor-Brown and Alejandro Garcia) The Haworth Press, Inc., 1999, pp. xiii-xv. Single or multiple copies of this article are available for a fee from The Haworth Document Delivery Service [1-800-342-9678, 9:00 a.m. - 5:00 p.m. (EST). E-mail address: getinfo@ haworthpressinc.com].

© 1999 by The Haworth Press, Inc. All rights reserved.

probability of poverty, substance abuse, and family dysfunction. These families are also more likely to be African American or Latino and facing racism, as well as the societal fear and discrimination that accompany the disease. The rapid rise of the disease–especially among African-American and Latino women and children–needs to be addressed with humanity, sensitivity, and ethnic-competent interventions at our disposal.

Living in a family in which a family member is HIV-infected has profound psychological effects on the child or adolescent. Having to face the mortality of a family member also confronts youth with their own mortality, and some cope with this by engaging in risky behavior which may result in the youth also becoming HIV infected. Recently a 13-year-old in an HIV-affected family was hospitalized for treatment of advanced gonorrhea. This young man had avoided treatment despite excruciatingly painful symptoms. This delay resulted in severe and irreversible health consequences. The reasons for the individual's refusal to seek treatment may rest on his fear of HIV disease or may be part of a self-destructive behavioral pattern. Lack of education about the disease and its prevention may be part of the problem. Separate from HIV, many find it difficult to talk with children about sexual and drug behaviors. HIV+ parents are further challenged by their own experiences of engaging in risk behaviors that resulted in their contracting HIV disease. Too often, shame and guilt prevent a parent from imparting in a meaningful way the necessary information regarding risk behaviors. Equally, the neighborhoods of these youth may contribute to risk due to poverty, drug dealing and limited resources. The inability or unwillingness of the family and neighborhood to provide support may also contribute to this phenomenon.

Researchers and mental health practitioners are faced with the dilemma of studying children and youth in HIV-infected families and providing recommendations on how to assist these individuals in resisting risky behaviors. Providing directions on support for these vulnerable individuals in the face of this chronic disease or death, poverty, drug abuse, and racism, as well as the tribulations that accompany adolescence, is a major challenge. Society needs to know how children and adolescents are surviving in these difficult situations and why some are doing less well than others.

American society needs to recognize that these children and adolescents will grow up to be part of our adult society. We need to insure that they grow up to be healthy, productive members of our society. The degree of their future contributions to this society will depend on how well we have responded to the crises they are confronting at this challenging time in their lives.

Susan Taylor-Brown
Alejandro Garcia

Introduction

Gary A. Lloyd

It is a commonplace that social stigma attaches to people with HIV disease, those who are affected by HIV/AIDS, and the programs which attempt to serve them. In the early days of the pandemic, some of us thought that with time and education the need to separate and stigmatize would lose intensity. History, demography, and epidemiology have, of course, proven such optimism to be sorely misplaced. As the articles here testify, stigma is a part of the every day social reality for HIV-affected children and their families who, in an allegedly child-oriented society, might be expected instead to benefit from social support.

· The needs and issues of HIV-affected children and their mothers and families have been addressed in the enormous and still growing literature on psychosocial dimensions of HIV disease. Still, given the well-known and observable demographic trends, we know too little. This fine collection of research studies both expands our knowledge and informs us of how much more we need to know.

Although each of these articles focuses on the needs of HIV-affected children, the methodologies, perspectives, and conclusions are diverse. Taken altogether, however, they speak as one voice in articulating fundamental and enduring realities of the majority of children and mothers who are affected by HIV disease: they are apt to be poor, people of color, living in substandard housing and subject to discrimination and social isolation. This demographic portrait is well-known.

Gary A. Lloyd, PhD, ACSW, DSW, is Professor Emeritus, Tulane University School of Social Work.

[Haworth co-indexing entry note]: "Introduction." Lloyd, Gary A. Co-published simultaneously in *Journal of HIV/AIDS Prevention & Education for Adolescents & Children* (The Haworth Press, Inc.) Vol. 3, No. 1/2, 1999, pp. 1-4; and: *HIV Affected and Vulnerable Youth: Prevention Issues and Approaches* (ed: Susan Taylor-Brown and Alejandro Garcia) The Haworth Press, Inc., 1999, pp. 1-4. Single or multiple copies of this article are available for a fee from The Haworth Document Delivery Service [1-800-342-9678, 9:00 a.m. - 5:00 p.m. (EST). E-mail address: getinfo@haworthpressinc.com].

© 1999 by The Haworth Press, Inc. All rights reserved.

Not so widely reported elsewhere as in these studies are the multiple losses experienced by women and children because of infection, crime, and substance abuse. These multiple, often environmentally rooted, losses can and do exacerbate the series of anticipated and actual losses from HIV disease.

Despite stigma and multiple losses, and despite the physical and social intensity of this disease, many children and their families manage to sustain themselves. The authors of these articles stress the ubiquity of strength and resilience even when the odds are very bad and worsening. Without ignoring the realities of family instability, personal and social barriers to obtaining or complying with treatment, substance abuse and disorganization, or the need for secrecy and fears about revealing HIV status, most of these authors find extraordinary capacities for coping. The strategies adopted by these infected mothers for themselves and their children may not be congruent with textbook theory but, as Mason and Korr observe, traditional models of coping behaviors need to be questioned.

Professionals in AIDS care may be as prone as other social service workers to ignore resilience and strength because those qualities are unexpected, or their manifestations do not fit with received wisdom about powerlessness and helplessness in HIV/AIDS-affected families. Certainly, the lives of HIV-affected children and their families are not tidy. They do not lend themselves to study through elegant and linear methodologies. These are lives characterized by resilience and complexity which, as Wiener et al. point out, are explainable only in models of non-linear development focusing on changing and uneven coping patterns of children over time.

Virtually from the outset of the pandemic, established mental health and social service agencies have been found wanting by many professionals and volunteers in AIDS care. Gilbert reflects some continuing concerns about the attitudes, values, and experiences of social service staffs which limit their understanding of HIV positive women and their children. She points out as well that women were ignored for years, or were viewed in the shadow of their children. Draimin et al. call for multiple and adaptive service models. Given the complexities of the lives and circumstances of HIV-affected children and their mothers, social service and AIDS care agencies hoping to provide adequate support to children and their mothers require constant renewal of information and staff energy. One wonders how frequently that renewal actually takes place, or is even thought about, in large child protection agencies with staff members largely uninformed about the effects of HIV disease on women and children, particularly those who are impoverished, stigmatized, and isolated. Meehan and Cranston advocate for legal rights of adolescents to obtain services without parental or guardian consent. Whether advocacy for such a position will come from even the more advanced AIDS care or mental health agencies is questionable. Political considerations are inescapable in implementing strategies such as those described by Ward and Waters which are required to prevent HIV infection in adolescents. In a population not highly motivated for self-protection, they raise enduring, and still unresolved issues, about how to stimulate behavior change in hopeless adolescents and adults. Issues of legal rights and prevention are not new, but they often become lost in political debates on parental rights or morality.

Custody of HIV affected children perhaps has been the issue most discussed in the press and by policy makers since the onset of the epidemic. Experience has taught service providers and volunteers that decisions about guardianship and custody are frequently delayed and often "irrational" in the view of professionals charged with child protection. What appears to be irrationality or denial, however, might in fact reflect the reality of overwhelmed mothers who, as Gilbert points out, are unable to obtain care for themselves and their children. Mason and Korr remark on the fact that decision making is often influenced by lack of prior successes. They also point out that women often have a smaller network of supporters than do men.

These studies stimulate thinking about what mental health professionals need to know to do their jobs effectively, and to serve people, particularly disenfranchised mothers and their children, who are affected by a stigmatizing infection and disease. Theories based in linear thinking and certainty do not have much utility for understanding or intervening in problems inherent in an episodic disease process. Wiener points out, for example, that HIV positive children may actually exhibit relatively stable functioning and resilience in coping with their health, but have difficulties in other aspects of their lives.

The HIV literature is full of studies, reports, and polemics which reaffirm ideas and practice approaches grounded in experience and tested over time. Those are often valuable as affirmations of what is possible and useful. The studies reported here go beyond what we know, or even what we need to know. They move us to think anew about issues and interventions connected to both the plight and the strengths of rapidly growing numbers of children and women affected by HIV/AIDS. Questions about just how to develop and deliver new services, while assuring that staff members have the most current knowledge and resources for renewal, may be only partially answerable. Faced with uncertainty, we can choose to be comfortable with what we know works, or we can begin to explore how to clarify and illuminate the areas of uncertainty. A challenge to mental health professionals and AIDS care workers is to conduct our practice with the same degree of resiliency and adaptability as these authors found in so many children, women, and families affected by HIV disease.

My Brother

Lauren Wall

I love him
I care for him
He is my brother

I worry about him
I fear for him
He is my brother

There are lots like him
And many are dying
And so is my brother.

It's all over the news
In papers and on T.V.
About kids like my brother

I used to live in fear
of others finding out
About my brother

We told the school
the community and press
About my brother

Lauren Wall (age 10) wrote this poem during a session with Dr. Lori Wiener at the National Institute of Health.

[Haworth co-indexing entry note]: "My Brother." Wall, Lauren. Co-published simultaneously in *Journal of HIV/AIDS Prevention & Education for Adolescents & Children* (The Haworth Press, Inc.) Vol. 3, No. 1/2, 1999, pp. 5-6; and: *HIV Affected and Vulnerable Youth: Prevention Issues and Approaches* (ed: Susan Taylor-Brown and Alejandro Garcia) The Haworth Press, Inc., 1999, pp. 5-6. Single or multiple copies of this article are available for a fee from The Haworth Document Delivery Service [1-800-342-9678, 9:00 a.m. - 5:00 p.m. (EST). E-mail address: getinfo@haworthpressinc.com].

© 1999 by The Haworth Press, Inc. All rights reserved. 5

I live in less fear
and have more friends
And so does my brother

I still live in fear
about the course of this disease
And the loss of my brother

I live each day
loving him so
He is my brother.

The Courage of a Woman

Lynette Logan

In 1985 a twenty-seven-year-old woman, named Barbara, sat in a hospital room, crying her eyes out. Barbara had just given birth to a lovely baby boy. Her son was a little underweight, but to the natural eye he was a normal baby. This was not the case, Barbara's baby was terminally ill. She had just found out she was infected with HIV, and had passed it on to her son. This seriously grieved Barbara. She had two daughters and a newborn son to take care of.

When Barbara left the hospital with her son, she had no idea what she was going to do. For the next few years Barbara went on with her life, trying to ignore reality. She told almost no one about her ordeal, especially her family. Barbara's husband was killed two years after she and her son were diagnosed with HIV. Barbara felt she had no one to talk to so she kept her burden to herself.

As the years went by Barbara was finding it hard to do the things she usually did. Her and her son were making lots of hospital visits. Sometimes they were sick for weeks or even months. Barbara's two daughters were healthy, but they were growing up and couldn't be kept in the dark much longer.

Barbara decided to tell her daughters the truth about her and their brother's disease. She kept it between her and them. Barbara was very afraid of what her friends and family would think about her situation. She didn't want to worry or upset them.

This essay was written by Lynette for her high school English class (March 13, 1997).

[Haworth co-indexing entry note]: "The Courage of a Woman." Logan, Lynette. Co-published simultaneously in *Journal of HIV/AIDS Prevention & Education for Adolescents & Children* (The Haworth Press, Inc.) Vol. 3, No. 1/2, 1999, pp. 7-8; and: *HIV Affected and Vulnerable Youth: Prevention Issues and Approaches* (ed: Susan Taylor-Brown and Alejandro Garcia) The Haworth Press, Inc., 1999, pp. 7-8. Single or multiple copies of this article are available for a fee from The Haworth Document Delivery Service [1-800-342-9678, 9:00 a.m. - 5:00 p.m. (EST). E-mail address: getinfo@haworthpressinc. com].

© 1999 by The Haworth Press, Inc. All rights reserved.

As the years went on and her illness progressed, Barbara found it hard for her to take care of herself and her children. Barbara married her longtime friend John. John loved Barbara and her kids, but wasn't much help to Barbara in her situation. She and John soon separated.

Once again it was just Barbara and her children. Barbara continued to get sick and had to be hospitalized. She felt this an opportune time to let her friends and family in on the fact that she and her son were ill. They took it very hard, but eventually gave their support. Now that Barbara had emotional help her burden wasn't so heavy. She decided to speak out about her disease and help other people. Whenever she was healthy enough Barbara educated others about HIV, starting with her children.

After a while Barbara developed A.I.D.S. A short while after this Barbara had a tough decision to make. Barbara had to arrange things for her children to be taken care of, after she passed away. Barbara loved her children enough to find them a home where they would be happy and well taken care of. She wanted to make this very easy for her children, so she explained everything to them, and slowly passed their well being over to a close friend of hers.

By the time Barbara was too ill to take care of herself, her children were safely being cared for. It was very hard for Barbara to give up her motherly duties. She laid her motherly pride down for the love of her children.

Barbara passed away in July of 1996. Due to her brave efforts to prepare for her children, they are doing well. Her sick son is at a time in his life where his health is stable. He is now able to be a typical eleven year-old. Barbara's two daughters are both doing fine for themselves. One is fifteen and the other is twenty. They both lead normal lives in the memory of their mother.

If Barbara hadn't prepared for the lives of her children, they would live in turmoil. In her thirty-eight years of life, Barbara Logan showed the world the courage of a woman.

When I Think of AIDS

Takiya S. McClain

When I think of AIDS and its impact on my life,
I can't help but to think of my father.
This disease ripped out all the dark secrets of his life,
interruption and dependence became routine,
and through it all he survived.
In my own way, I will try to explain my feelings towards this illness,
how I came to terms with these feelings,
and how I plan to make the best of what it left me.

Alone, not afraid

To be honest, I always thought that my father would get HIV. You see, the life he led guaranteed him a one way ticket right to AIDS, my father was a drug-addict. I've always thought that I would be afraid of something that could take any and everything from you, but when I met AIDS, I knew different. After my dad was infected, he became the father he should have been, the husband he wanted to be, and the man he always was. You see, my father didn't change, he got better. First, AIDS takes over your life, mind, body, and soul, leaves you vulnerable, and then makes you the person you always wanted to be. Then it

---

This poem was written by Takiya in an HIV/AIDS seminar at Syracuse University where she was studying to become a nurse (September 11, 1996).

[Haworth co-indexing entry note]: "When I Think of AIDS." McClain, Takiya S. Co-published simultaneously in *Journal of HIV/AIDS Prevention & Education for Adolescents & Children* (The Haworth Press, Inc.) Vol. 3, No. 1/2, 1999, pp. 9-11; and: *HIV Affected and Vulnerable Youth: Prevention Issues and Approaches* (ed: Susan Taylor-Brown and Alejandro Garcia) The Haworth Press, Inc., 1999, pp. 9-11. Single or multiple copies of this article are available for a fee from The Haworth Document Delivery Service [1-800-342-9678, 9:00 a.m. - 5:00 p.m. (EST). E-mail address: getinfo@haworthpressinc. com].

© 1999 by The Haworth Press, Inc. All rights reserved.

scoops you up and takes from you all the people you love and who love you. Once you've met AIDS, you realize that it doesn't make you afraid, it just leaves you alone.

Interruption

AIDS interrupts all aspects of your life. It allows you to feel feelings that become confusing and hard to describe. You feel:

- Hurt–"Why is this happening?"
- Sad–"I don't want my daddy to die."
- Happy–"Our relationship has gotten better."

I felt all of these feelings, all at the same time, and all for the same person. Sometimes I wonder, how I ever made it with a smile on my face. People never seemed to think that any thing was wrong in my life, but there was an immeasurable interruption in my life, my daddy was dying and there was nothing I could do about it. All I could do was sit in my room and stare at the cool white walls and cry.

Dependence

I began to feel like AIDS was taking over my life, as my father's condition got worse, I began to lose it more and more. I needed someone, somebody to help me help myself. I began to reach out to my peers and advisors. I always thought that I would be strong enough to "be all right," but that's how much AIDS takes from you. I remember my dad writing me on the pad he used in the hospital, ". . . it will take your life if you let it." It was then that I realized that I had to fight AIDS with all that I had, I had to continue my daddy's struggle and beat this thing.

Survival

Now that I'm a survivor of AIDS, I have put on my whole armor, and I'm ready for warfare. AIDS has taken away someone that meant the world to me, and I'm ready to get my revenge.

AFTERWORD

This course, AIDS: Response to the Pandemic, will train me to be the soldier I need to be and will give me the weapons I need in my fight with AIDS. I thought I knew all I needed to know about AIDS, but I was wrong. In the short time that I've been in training, I've learned so much more. I hope that I will have the will, strength, and wisdom to continue in my fight against AIDS, with the sweet memory of my father dear to my heart.

Longitudinal Study
of Psychological Distress Symptoms
in HIV-Infected, School-Aged Children

Lori Wiener
Haven Battles
Kristin A. Riekert

SUMMARY. Despite the growing numbers of HIV-infected school-aged children, we know very little about the mental health status of this group. This longitudinal study examined the frequency of psychological distress symptoms in HIV-infected children between the ages of 6 and 11 years at three time points over a period of two and one-half years. Children were assessed using the Dominic, a pictorial instrument that assesses for 7 psychological distress symptoms of childhood. In addition, family and demographic variables were collected at Time 1. Children were found to be relatively well-adjusted, with low to moderate incidence of psychological distress. While there were no significant changes in frequency of psychological distress symptoms from Time 1 to Time 3, the prevalence of overanxious and depressive symptomatology increased over time. Implications for clinical practice and future research will be discussed. *[Article copies available for a fee from The Haworth Document Delivery Service: 1-800-342-9678. E-mail address: getinfo@haworthpressinc.com]*

Lori Wiener, PhD, ACSW, is Coordinator, Pediatric HIV Psychosocial Support Program, HIV/AIDS Malignancy Branch, National Cancer Institute, 9000 Rockville Pike, Building 10/Room 13N240, Bethesda, MD 20892.

Haven Battles, MPhil, is Research Associate, HIV/AIDS Malignancy Branch, National Cancer Institute, 9000 Rockville Pike, Building 10/Room 13N240, Bethesda, MD 20892.

Kristin A. Riekert, MA, is a graduate student, Department of Psychology, Case Western Reserve University, 10900 Euclid Avenue, Cleveland, OH 44106.

[Haworth co-indexing entry note]: "Longitudinal Study of Psychological Distress Symptoms in HIV-Infected, School-Aged Children." Wiener, Lori, Haven Battles, and Kristin A. Riekert. Co-published simultaneously in *Journal of HIV/AIDS Prevention & Education for Adolescents & Children* (The Haworth Press, Inc.) Vol. 3, No. 1/2, 1999, pp. 13-36; and: *HIV Affected and Vulnerable Youth: Prevention Issues and Approaches* (ed: Susan Taylor-Brown and Alejandro Garcia) The Haworth Press, Inc., 1999, pp. 13-36. Single or multiple copies of this article are available for a fee from The Haworth Document Delivery Service [1-800-342-9678, 9:00 a.m. - 5:00 p.m. (EST). E-mail address: getinfo@haworthpressinc.com].

KEYWORDS. HIV-infected children, psychological distress, anxiety, depression, adjustment

INTRODUCTION

As of June, 1997, 7,902 children aged 13 and under were diagnosed with AIDS in the US (CDC, 1997). As the number of HIV-infected women of child-bearing age rises (CDC, 1997), the number of exposed infants being born also increases. While some HIV-infected children die within the first few years of life, a substantial number of others have survived early childhood and are living well into adolescence and young adulthood. Recent studies have contributed to the knowledge base regarding survival rates of HIV-infected children (Grubman et al., 1995; Tovo et al., 1992), one of whom (Tovo et al., 1992) indicated that over 49.5% of these children survive for more than 9 years. Since mortality is no longer perceived to be imminent, researchers are slowly beginning to examine the psychological needs of this pediatric population.

PREVALENCE OF ADJUSTMENT PROBLEMS

It has been estimated that children with a chronic illness have a risk for adjustment problems that is 1.5 to 3 times greater than their healthy peers (Pless, 1984). In a large-scale epidemiological study, Cadman, Boyle, Szatmari, and Offord (1987) found that 33% of children with a chronic physical condition could be diagnosed with at least one DSM-III disorder compared to 14% of the physically healthy children. Thompson, Hodges, and Hamlett (1990) found that 58% of children with cystic fibrosis, compared to 23% of nonreferred children and 77% of psychiatrically referred children met criteria for a major DSM-III diagnosis. The children with cystic fibrosis were similar to the nonreferred children except in terms of worries, poor self-image, and anxiety, where their symptom levels were comparable to that of the psychiatrically referred children. Consistent with other pediatric chronic illness (Thompson & Gustafson, 1996), previous studies have found that children with HIV are at risk for internalizing psychological adjustment problems, particularly anxiety disorders (Bussing &

Burket, 1993; Havens, Whitaker, Feldman & Ehrhardt, 1994; Hooper, Whitt, Tennison, Burchinal, Gold, and Hall, 1993; Riekert, Wiener, Battles, & Drotar, in press).

Few studies, however, have been completed which specifically look at psychological adjustment of HIV-infected children. Havens, Whitaker, Feldman, and Ehrhardt (1994) compared drug exposed HIV-infected children living with foster families with seroreverted children and non-HIV-exposed children who were also drug exposed and living with foster families. They found a high rate of psychiatric morbidity, especially rates of disruptive behaviors, in all three groups. These high rates were attributed to the common background factors in the groups, such as drug exposure. They also found that the HIV-infected children were experiencing higher levels of subjective distress, in the form of anxiety, than the two comparative groups on both parent report and self-report instruments. This increased anxiety appeared to be independent of their knowledge of their HIV status.

Contrary to the above results, a second study (Bose et al., 1994) found that on self-report measures HIV-infected children reported significantly less depression and anxiety and had a more positive self-concept than normal, healthy children based on test norms. Parent reports agreed with the child reports except that they indicated the presence of moderate adjustment problems. Several demographic variables differentiated the two samples which may account for the discrepancy. For example, Bose et al.'s children were older, the majority had acquired HIV through transfusion, lived in two-parent families, and knew their diagnosis. In light of these differences, we felt that it was essential to evaluate the influences of various mediating variables on the presence or absence of psychological disturbances in school-aged, HIV-infected children.

The research that has been done suggests that, while simply having a chronic illness such as HIV increases a child's risk for mental health and adjustment problems, one cannot assume that a child with HIV will always experience poor psychological adjustment. Much of the literature, particularly the studies of children with HIV, are limited because they tend to use behavior problem checklists to measure adjustment which do not provide diagnostic information (Wallander & Thompson, 1995). Moreover, when children's self-reports of their psychological adjustment are obtained, they are often assessed using measures that exclusively examine internalizing problems, such as depression and anxiety (Thompson & Gustafson, 1996). By only assessing internalizing symptoms, essential information about the complete picture of the child's psychological adjustment remains unknown. Therefore, it is important to examine the children's overall behavioral adjustment and include an assessment of both internalizing and externalizing disorders.

STABILITY OF ADJUSTMENT PROBLEMS

To truly understand the development prospective of adjustment to chronic illness, one must consider the changes in symptom presentation over time (Thompson & Gustafson 1996). Despite this recognition, relatively few longitudinal studies have been conducted that have examined the change in the frequency and types of adjustment problems over time. Thompson and colleagues have presented longitudinal adjustment data for children with cystic fibrosis and sickle cell disease (Thompson, Gil, Keith, Gustafson, George, & Kinney, 1994; Thompson, Gustafson, George, & Spock, 1994).

In the sample of 41 children with cystic fibrosis between the ages of seven and fourteen years, Thompson, Gustafson et al. (1994) found that the prevalence of child-reported adjustment problems in terms of DSM-III diagnoses was nearly identical at the initial assessment (63%) and at a 12-month follow-up (61%). When examining the stability of adjustment at the individual level, they found that 49% of the children had stable poor adjustment, 24% had stable good adjustment, but 27% changed classification over time. Anxiety diagnoses and oppositional defiant disorder were the most frequent diagnoses at both time periods. There was little congruence, however, in individuals' specific diagnoses from time one to time two assessment. Mother-reported data was similar with consistent prevalence rates of adjustment problems being reported at both time points (63 initial, 58% follow-up). According to the mother, fifty-four percent reported stable poor adjustment, 32% had stable good adjustment, and 15% reported a change in classification between the two time points. Again, there was a relatively low rate of congruence in child's specific diagnoses at the two assessments.

Similar results were found in a sample of 35 children (aged 7-14 years) with sickle cell disease (Thompson, Gil et al., 1994). Child-reported prevalence rate of adjustment problems was 49% at both the initial assessment and at a 10-month follow-up. At the individual level, however, 40% of the children changed classification over the 10-month follow-up. Twenty-nine percent had stable poor classification and 31% had stable good classification. Although anxiety diagnoses were the most frequent at both time points, there was little congruence in children's specific diagnoses over time. Mother-reported prevalence rates of adjustment were stable over time (60% initial, 69% follow-up). Thirty-one percent of mothers reported a change in adjustment classification, 49% reported stable poor adjustment, and 20% reported stable good psychological adjustment. Again, there was little congruence in the specific diagnoses from time one to time two.

CORRELATES OF PSYCHOLOGICAL ADJUSTMENT

In order to identify, understand, and treat the subset of children with chronic illnesses who are experiencing poor psychological adjustment, research has examined a variety of correlates to adjustment. Typically, the correlates of psychological adjustment are organized along three dimensions: condition parameters, child parameters, and social-ecological parameters. These dimensions have been reviewed extensively elsewhere (see Lavigne & Faier-Routman, 1993; Thompson & Gustafson, 1996; Wallander & Thompson, 1995) and therefore will be briefly summarized here and discussed as they relate to HIV-infection.

Condition/Disease Parameters

Condition Type. Typically, there are no differences in psychological adjustment found between different physical illnesses. However, more behavioral problems are typically found among children with conditions affecting the brain than among children with conditions not involving the brain (Austin & Huberty, 1993; Breslau, 1985; Walker, Ortiz-Valdes, & Newbrough, 1989). HIV has been shown to have a devastating effect on infected children's central nervous system (Civitello et al., 1993; Englund et al., 1996). Estimates based on samples observed in the last decade suggest that 50% of children with HIV-1 disease have evidence of HIV-related CNS abnormality (from mild to severe) with the lowest rates being in adolescents (33%) and the highest rates (from 65 to 75%) being infants (Butler et al., 1991; Chase et al., 1995; Englund et al., 1996). However, only 13% may display progressive encephalopathy, the most severe form of CNS disease in children (Blanche, Mayaux et al., 1994; European Collaborative Study, 1990; Lobato et al., 1995). As a result of CNS abnormalities, several social and emotional changes have been noted. These changes include decreased level of interaction and communication with others, apathy, flattened affect, and the inability to complete tasks or show goal-directed behavior (Wiener, Fair, & Pizzo, 1993; Moss et al., 1994 Roelofs, Wolters et al., 1996; Englund et al., 1996). Because of the presence of neurological impairment, we expect to find a high prevalence of poor psychological adjustment (Wiener et al., in press).

Condition Severity. Some studies have found that a longer disease duration and/or greater illness severity were related to more adjustment problems (Daniels, Moos, Billings, & Miller, 1987; Steinhausen, Schindler, & Stephan, 1983) and others have found that disease severity has little or no relationship to an ill child's psychological dysfunction (Billings, Moos, Miller, & Gottlieb, 1987; Thompson, Gustafson, Hamlett, & Spock, 1992; Wallander & Thompson, 1995). The findings of Lavigne and Faier-Routman's (1993) meta-analysis provides support for the contributions of the severity of the child's illness to adjustment. This study, however, likely confounded illness severity with condition type. In studies of children infected with HIV, Bose et al. (1994) and Riekert et al. (in press) found that illness severity, operationalized as CD4%, was not significantly correlated with child report of depression or trait anxiety symptoms. When looking at parent report of symptoms, Bose et al. found that CD4% was negatively correlated with anxiety symptoms, but was not correlated with conduct disorder or hyperactivity. Riekert et al., did not find a correlation between parent-reported anxious/depressed symptoms and CD4%. Due to the inconsistency of results of the previous studies, we have included a measure of illness severity, CD4%, in the current study.

Disease Variables

Children with HIV/AIDS bring into the picture another disease variable, route of transmission, which may influence results when comparing children within the diagnosis of HIV. HIV-infected children are typically infected vertically (mother-to-child) (91%), through a hemophilia-related transfusion (3%), or through transfusion of blood components or tissue (5%) (CDC, 1997). Each mode brings with it characteristics which distinguish it from the others and which may have a significant influence upon a child's mental health status. For example, many children who are infected perinatally have mothers who used drugs during pregnancy. Higher rates of behavior disorders have been noted in non-HIV-infected, drug-exposed children (Davis et al., 1992; Rodning, Beckwith, & Howard, 1989). It may be difficult to separate the effects of drug exposure from psychological problems which may arise from the influence of the HIV-infection. In addition, if children are living with their biological parents, they must deal with multiple family members being infected with HIV. If their biological parents have died or are not able to care for them (due to their own illness or individual circumstances), they have the additional challenge of grieving the loss of a parent(s) while adjusting to a new family within either an extended family members', a foster, or an adoptive home.

Children with hemophilia have a different set of characteristics. For example, these children were faced with living with a chronic illness even before their HIV diagnosis. Recent research suggests that living with the dual diagnoses of hemophilia and HIV can cause distress for both the child (Brown, Schultz, & Gragg, 1995) and parent (Drotar, Agle, Eckl, & Thompson, 1995). It is not clear whether one diagnosis overshadows the other, if there is an additive effect in which the child is at double the risk for psychological disturbance, or if living with hemophilia has strengthened the child's coping skills so that adjustment to the HIV diagnosis is facilitated.

Children who acquired HIV through a regular blood transfusion are similar to hemophilia-acquired children in that they have often already faced a life-threatening event such as premature birth, leukemia, or a major cardiac impairment that necessitated a transfusion. Clinical observation has suggested that these families sometimes develop a sense of mistrust toward the medical establishment because the treatment they believed would help save their child's life later turned out to infect them with a terminal illness. Parents may also experience guilt at not insisting that their own blood be transfused to the child or anger over not having been offered that option (Wiener & Septimus, 1994).

Child Parameters

Gender. There is little consensus about the role of gender in a child's psychological adjustment. Typically, no gender differences have been reported except for Wallander et al. (1988), who found that boys scored higher on the Externalizing Behavior Problems scale of the Child Behavior Checklist. It has been suggested that the magnitude of the contribution is dependent upon who is reporting the child's adjustment (Wallander & Thompson, 1995). When adjustment is assessed by child-report, girls report more symptoms of distress than boys (e.g., Ryan & Morrow, 1986; Thompson et al., 1992). In a study of children with HIV, Riekert et al. (in press) found that girls reported significantly more trait anxiety and separation anxiety symptoms than boys, but similar depressive symptoms. Because of the potential for gender differences, we have included gender as an independent variable in the current study.

Age. Studies are fairly consistent across conditions with regard to a lack of an age effect on psychological adjustment (Wallander & Thompson, 1995), although some exceptions have been noted (e.g., Thompson et al., 1990). These studies, however, have been cross-sectional. Longitudinal investigations are necessary to accurately assess the influence of age on adjustment (Thompson & Gustafson, 1996). In a cross-sectional study of children with HIV, Riekert et al. (in press) found that younger children reported significantly more separation anxiety symptoms. There were no age differences on depressive or trait-anxiety symptoms. Parents of older children, however, reported more anxious/depressed symptoms for older children. As a result of the above findings and Thompson and Gustafson's comments regarding the lack of longitudinal information about the influence of age on adjustment, we have included age as an independent variable in the present study.

Social-Ecological Parameters

Socioeconomic Status. Lower SES has consistently been associated with an increased rate of psychological adjustment problems among mental health populations. The relationship has not consistently been found in the pediatric chronic illness literature, perhaps because a consistent measure of SES has not been used (Thompson & Gustafson, 1996). Wallander et al. (1988) found that even when they controlled for SES, the chronically ill children still had significantly higher Externalizing and Internalizing Behavior Problem scale scores compared to a normative sample. In a study of children with HIV, Riekert et al. (in press) found no correlation between income and parent-report of anxious/depressed symptoms or child-report of depressive or trait anxiety symptoms. A negative correlation between income and child-report of separation anxiety symptoms, however, was found. Wallander and Thompson (1995) recommends that SES always be considered as a potential contributor to the adjustment of children with chronic illness. Within the pediatric HIV population, affected families are often single-parent families, have limited education and economic resources, and lack medical insurance (The Working Group, 1996).

Family Functioning. Unlike virtually any other childhood illness today, HIV presents families with unique social stresses, including public fear and ignorance regarding the nature and transmission of HIV, discrimination, isolation, social ostracism, stigma, and fear of physical and mental disability. HIV also challenges the integrity of the family unit as multiple family members are often infected. HIV/AIDS disproportionately affects minorities; over 80% of HIV-infected children are from minority backgrounds (CDC, 1997). While there is no single portrait of an HIV-infected child, they are, in large measure, children who have already experienced the burdens of poverty, seen the effects of substance abuse and violence, and endured many other types of loss and trauma in their families (Working Committee of HIV, AIDS & families, 1996). Frequently, these families must deal with issues stemming from drug abuse, poverty, disclosure of HIV status, and physical illness while simultaneously planning for the future of their well children who will be orphaned. Therefore, even without evidence of neurologic involvement, attentional difficulties, hyperactivity, depression, and anxiety may be present due to a parent's death, chaotic family environments, poverty, or exposure to toxic substances (Barkley, 1990).

There is also strong support for the role of family functioning in child psychological adjustment across of a number of different conditions (Thompson & Gustafson, 1996; Daniels et al., 1987). Family functioning is considered to have both a direct and indirect influence on adjustment. Measures of family functioning that reflect supportive family relationships, such as family cohesion, tend to be related to better psychological adjustment, while measures of problematic family qualities (e.g., conflict) tend to be related to poorer psychological adjustment (Drotar, 1997). Pless, Roghmann, and Haggerty (1972) found that chronically ill children from poorly functioning families were at greater risk for developing psychological adjustment problems than their healthy counterparts. These problems can be emotional, for example, depression has been related to family functioning (Shulman et al., 1991), or they can be behavioral. Although family functioning has been found to be a strong correlate with child psychological adjustment, it has not been studied in pediatric HIV populations. Therefore, we have included family functioning as an independent variable.

Parental Adjustment

While there have been some non-significant findings (e.g., Kovacs et al., 1986), there is considerable support for a positive relationship between parental depression and mother-reported child adjustment (Wallander & Thompson, 1995). It has been suggested that this relationship reflects maternal report bias, however, some studies have found that children's reports of their own psychological symptoms are related to maternal psychological symptoms (e.g., Thompson et al., 1992; Walker et al., 1989). In a study of children with HIV, Riekert et al. (in press) found that parental depression and trait anxiety symptoms were positively correlated with their report of their child's anxious/depressed symptoms, but were not significantly correlated with the child's report of psychological distress (e.g., depressive, trait anxiety, and separation anxiety symptoms). We have included parental adjustment as an independent variable in the current study to further study the relationship between parental and child adjustment.

THE PRESENT STUDY

The current study was designed to advance scientific knowledge about the psychological adjustment of children with HIV along several constructs. This longitudinal study of a sample of children with HIV seen at a hospital-based clinic examines the frequency of psychological distress symptoms in children between the ages of 6 and 11 years. To our knowledge, it is the first to longitudinally examine the prevalence of adjustment problem symptoms in children with HIV-infection. By following the sample of children over a two-and-a-half year period, we had the opportunity to examine the stability of symptoms associated with psychological adjustment problems. Furthermore, with the exception of one study, which utilized the same sample to examine the relationship between parent and child reports of distress (Riekert et al., in press), no studies have investigated the psychological correlates typically found to be associated with psychological adjustment across a number of different medical conditions. By delineating the correlates of adjustment, the goal of this study was to advance knowledge about the process of adjustment as well as guide treatment and prevention interventions for children with HIV-infection. Since highly structured interviews may not be appropriate for use with younger children (Schwab-Stone et al., 1994), in this study, children were assessed at three separate time points using the "Dominic," a valid and reliable cartoon-like instrument designed to study the mental health status of children aged 6-11. Information on demographics, family environment, parental psychological functioning and parent report of child's psychological functioning were also collected at Time 1.

METHODS

Participants

Seventy families of HIV-infected, school-aged children (ages 6-11) from the Pediatric Branch of the National Cancer Institute were asked to participate in the study. At Time 1, 64 of a total 70 families agreed to participate, resulting in a response rate of 91%. At Time 2 (6 months later), 50 children were assessed, and at Time 3 (18 months after Time 2) 49 children were interviewed. Forty-four families were retained in the final analysis, yielding a final response rate of 63%. Of the original 64 children, 7 died over the course of the study, 7 did not have scheduled appointments during at least one of the data collection periods, and due to a decline in neuropsychological skills, 1 lacked the cognitive abilities to complete the tasks. These 15 children, in addition to 5 that were dropped because of missing data, did not differ significantly in gender, ethnicity, SES, mode of transmission, parent gender, parent ethnicity, parent HIV status, prenatal drug exposure, parent's marital status, or relationship to parent (e.g., biological, foster, adoptive or extended) from the rest of the children.

The mean age of the children in this study at Time 1 was 8.2 years. Remaining demographic characteristics of both the children and caregivers are summarized in Table 1.

Procedure

Participants were approached by a social worker (LW) when they arrived for their clinic appointments and asked if they would be willing to participate in the study. If they agreed, an appointment was then scheduled to meet with an interviewer at some time during their visit to NCI. All measures were administered at Time 1 and the Dominic was re-administered at Times 2 and 3.

TABLE 1. Demographic characteristics of sample (n = 44).

Demographic trait		
Parent gender	Female	91%
	Male	9%
Child gender	Female	48%
	Male	52%
Parent ethnicity	Caucasian	76%
	African American	17%
	Hispanic	7%
Child ethnicity	Caucasian	59%
	African American	32%
	Hispanic	9%
Relationship to child		
	Biological	65%
	Foster/Adoptive	35%
Parent HIV serostatus		
	HIV −	79%
	HIV+	21%
Family Income		
	Less than $10,000	17%
	$10,000-$19,999	12%
	$20,000-$29,999	17%
	$30,000-$39,999	12%
	$40,000-$49,999	17%
	$50,000-$100,000	17%
	More than $100,000	7%
Child route of transmission		
	Vertical	75%
	Transfusion	23%
	Hemophilia	2%
Does child know diagnosis? (At time 1)		
	Yes	76%
	No	54%

Instruments (Time 1 Only)

The Child Behavior Checklist. The CBCL (Achenbach, 1991) obtains standardized information about behavioral problems. Parents complete the measure which provides both a total behavior problem score as well as scores for two second-order, or broad-band, factors labeled Internalizing and Externalizing. Symptoms of Internalizing problems include social withdrawal, somatic complaints, anxiety and depression whereas symptoms of externalizing problems refer to more disruptive behaviors such as delinquency, aggression, and hyperactivity. Internal consistency for normative samples ranges from .56 to .96 (Achenbach, 1991).

The Spielberger State-Trait Anxiety Inventory (Spielberger, 1983) was used to assess parental anxiety levels. The State Anxiety Scale and the Trait Anxiety Scale are each composed of 20 items on a 4 point Likert scale. In the State Anxiety Scale the subject is asked to indicate how he feels at this moment while in the Trait Anxiety Scale he is asked to respond how he generally feels. Watson and Clark (1984) documented the high correlation of the State-Trait Anxiety Inventory with many other anxiety scales. High test-retest reliability has been reported for trait anxiety with this questionnaire.

The Beck Depression Inventory (BDI-Beck, 1967) is a 21-item, self-report measure that assesses the frequency of depression in the caregiver. Average internal consistency was .85 for the six normative samples that Beck studied (Beck, 1987).

Family Environment Scale (FES-Moos and Moos, 1986) was completed by the primary caregiver and assesses ten aspects of the family environment. The sub-scales which are of most importance to this study include: the Cohesion scale, which assesses the degree of commitment, help and support members provide for one another; the Expressiveness scale, the extent to which members are encouraged to act openly and express feelings directly; the Conflict scale, the amount of openly expressed anger, aggression, and conflict among members; the Organization scale, the degree of importance ascribed by the family to clear organization and structure in planning family activities and responsibilities; and the Control scale, the extent to which set rules and procedures are used to run family life. All scales were developed on a theoretical-rational basis. The internal consistency (alpha > .6) and 2 month test-retest reliability (r > .7) are adequate for this scale (Moos & Moos, 1986).

The Health Status Questionnaire. This brief questionnaire was written by the principal investigator and was completed by the physician or nurse practitioner examining the child the day the child and caregiver completed the questionnaires. It obtains information regarding the most recent percent CD4 positive cells (T4%), subjective ratings of the child's health status, and degree of debilitation.

The Demographic Questionnaire. Data concerning parent and child characteristics were collected via parent self-report. The information collected included age, gender, socioeconomic status (SES), ethnicity, and questions specific to HIV such as route of transmission, whether the child knows his/her HIV diagnosis, and parental HIV-serostatus.

Instruments (Time 1, 2, and 3)

The Dominic (Valla, Bergeron, Bérubé, & Gaudet, 1994; Valla, Bergeron, Bidaut-Russell, St-Georges, & Gaudet, 1997) is a cartoon-based questionnaire designed to study the mental health status of children aged six to eleven. The drawings conveyed situations based on symptoms of the seven more prevalent diagnoses in the DSM-III-R Axis I: Attention Deficit Hyperactivity Disorder (ADHD), Conduct Disorder (CD), Oppositional Defiant Disorder (ODD), Major Depressive Disorder/Dysthymia (MDD), Separation Anxiety Disorder (SAD), Overanxious Disorder (OAD), and Simple Phobia (SPh). Children are shown a series of 97 cartoon drawings. In 89 of these, a child, "Dominic," is depicted exhibiting 95 symptoms covering 62 of the 66 DSM-III-R criteria included in these diagnoses. Mixed in with these are eight pictures of a smiling Dominic enjoying various activities. Children are asked to respond 'yes' they are like Dominic or 'no' they are not. The Dominic/Dominique character was designed to be interpreted as either a boy or girl to allow assessment of both genders. Internal consistency for each of the subscales ranged from .62 to .88 (Valla, Bergeron, Bérubé, & Gaudet, 1994) and from .80 to .90 for our sample.

RESULTS

Findings at Time 1

Demographics. Correlation analyses (see Table 2) and one way ANOVAs (see Table 3) (where independent variables were categorical) were run between the child's demographic characteristics and

TABLE 2. Matrix of significant correlations.

Correlation matrix of child's age and CD4% with psychological variables

	Child's Age r	CD4% r
SAD (Dominic)	− .37***	.31**
OAD (Dominic)		.46****
Sph (Dominic)	− .28*	
MDD (Dominic)	ns	.28*
Withdrawn (CBCL)	.31**	ns
Somatic (CBCL)	.31**	ns
Anxious/Depressed (CBCL)	.38***	ns
Internalizing (CBCL)	.38***	ns

Note: * = p < .10, ** = p < .05, *** = p < .01, **** = p < .005, ns = not significant

TABLE 3. F scores for ANOVAs of psychosocial and demographic variables at Time 1.

	Gender F	Route of Transmission F	P
SAD (Dominic)	5.76[1]**		
OAD (Dominic)	5.85[1]**		
SPh (Dominic)	8.92[1]****		
MDD (Dominic)	4.83[1]**		
Internalizing (CBCL)	ns		4.75[2]**

Note: * = p < .10, ** = p < .05, *** = p < .01, **** = p < .005, ns = not significant; [1]Boys scored higher than girls; [2]Children with transfusion- or hemophilia-acquired HIV scored higher than those with vertically acquired HIV.

results from the Dominic and the Child Behavior Checklist (CBCL) at Time 1. Child's age was negatively correlated with separation anxiety ($r = -.37$, $p < .01$) and simple phobia ($r = -.28$, $p < .10$) (from the Dominic Time 1) and positively associated with parent's report (CBCL) of withdrawn behavior ($r = .31$, $p < .05$), somatic complaints ($r = .31$, $p < .05$), anxiety/depression ($r = .38$, $p < .01$), and overall internalizing behavior ($r = .38$, $p < .01$). Boys were more likely to exhibit separation anxiety ($F = 5.76$, $p < .03$), overanxious disorder (F =

5.85, p < .02), simple phobia (F = 8.92, p < .005) and depression (F = 4.83, p < .04). Parents rated children (CBCL) with transfusion/hemophilia-acquired HIV as having more internalizing problems in general than those with vertically acquired HIV (F = 4.75, p < .02). Child's CD4% was positively associated with scores for separation anxiety (r = .31, p < .05), overanxious disorder (r = .46, p < .005), and depression (r = .28, p < .10) (Dominic). No significant differences in the psychological variables were found for child's awareness of his/her diagnosis.

Psychosocial Findings. Frequency of diagnosis according to the Child Behavior Checklist (from Time 1), and the Dominic (from Times 1, 2, & 3) are given in Tables 4 and 6, respectively. Means and standard deviations of the parents' Time 1 scores on the Beck Depression Inventory, the Spielberger State-Trait Anxiety Inventory and the Family Environment Scale can be found in Table 5.

The mean score on the Beck Depression Inventory was 10.1, which indicated that the caregivers in this sample scored in the mild to moderate range for depression. The women in this sample (n = 40) scored in the 71st percentile for state anxiety and the 69th percentile for trait anxiety, while the men (n = 4) scored in the 66th percentile for state and the 71st percentile for trait anxiety, according to published norms (Spielberger, 1983). Families also scored in normal ranges on Cohesion, Expressiveness, Conflict, Organization, and Control, according to published norms (Moos & Moos, 1986).

Results from the Family Environment Scale indicated that conflict was positively correlated with parental depression (r = .43, p < .01), parental trait anxiety (r = .47, p < .05), CBCL scores of anxiety/de-

TABLE 4. Number of children scoring in the normal, borderline, and clinical ranges on the CBCL at Time 1.

	Time 1		
	Normal	Borderline	Clinical
Withdrawn	85%	7%	7%
Somatic Complaints	62%	7%	31%
Anxious/Depressed	88%	7%	5%
Social Problems	93%	2%	5%
Thought Problems	95%	2%	2%
Attention Problems	95%	0%	5%
Delinquent Behavior	86%	7%	7%
Aggressive Behavior	88%	10%	2%

TABLE 5. Means and standard deviations of Parental measures at Time 1 (n = 42).

	Mean	S.D.
Beck Depression Inventory	10.1	8.5
State Anxiety	40.6	12.6
Trait Anxiety	39.3	10.9
Family Cohesion	6.6	2.3
Family Expressiveness	5.6	1.7
Family Conflict	3.3	1.9
Family Organization	6.0	2.3
Family Control	5.2	1.7

TABLE 6. Frequency of diagnosis according to the Dominic* at 3 time points (n = 44).

Disorder	Time 1	Time 2	Time 3
Separation Anxiety Disorder (SAD)	20%	9%	20%
Overanxious Disorder (OAD)	7%	2%	13%
Oppositional Defiant Disorder (ODD)	11%	5%	10%
Simple Phobia (SPh)	16%	7%	5%
Conduct Disorder (CD)	2%	2%	2%
Moor Depression/Dysthymia (MDD)	7%	5%	10%
Attention Deficit/Hyperactivity Disorder (ADHD)	9%	2%	15%

*The Dominic does not assess for frequency, duration, or onset of symptoms. Hence, these "diagnoses" are not referring to actual clinical diagnoses, but rather, they are an indication of the possible prevalence of these disorders in our sample.

pression (r = .54, p < .0005), internalizing (r = .43, p < .01), externalizing (r = .32, p < .05), and total behavior problems (r = .38, p < .05). Cohesion was negatively correlated with parental depression (r = −.42, p < .01), parental trait anxiety (r = −.42, p < .01), and CBCL anxiety/ depression (r = −.39, p < .01).

Longitudinal Analysis. Repeated measures ANOVA's including all three time points indicated that, according to the Dominic, there were no statistically significant changes in frequency of psychological distress symptoms over a period of 2 and one-half years.

Discussion and Clinical Implications

Prior studies examining the effect of HIV on a child's psychological functioning have presented a confusing picture. The differences have been attributed mainly to the demographic differences in the samples. One sample included HIV-infected drug-exposed children, all of whom were living in foster care and most of whom did not know their diagnosis (Havens et al., 1994). The other sample included older children, the majority of whom knew their diagnosis, had acquired the virus as a result of a contaminated blood transfusion, and who were living in two-parent families (Bose et al., 1994). This study attempted to bridge the earlier studies by studying a group of school-age children with varied demographic backgrounds at three time points over a two-year period of time.

The results of this study indicate that our sample of school-aged, HIV-infected children are exhibiting relatively stable psychological functioning. Psychological distress symptoms were only seen in a minority of our sample. Similar to both earlier studies, psychological distress appeared to be independent of children's knowledge of their HIV status. Severity of illness, whether rated by the child's care provider or analyzed according to the child's absolute T4 count, also did not predict psychological functioning. Vulnerability to psychological distress may be more related to a number of other variables which affect the child's life. These include the potential loss of one or both parents, siblings' HIV status, poverty, discrimination, ostracism, and the difficulty of coping with a life-threatening disease.

There were some trends that are worth noting. Symptoms of separation anxiety were found in 20% of our sample, a finding that is consistent with clinical observations of this patient population. Depressive symptomatology increased slightly over time (7%-10%). This is important to note, as the longer the child lives with HIV, the more losses they are likely to experience. The children also tended to report higher levels of psychological distress than their caregivers did. While discrepency betweeen child and caregiver report is described in the general and chronic illness literature (Achenbach, McConaughy, & Howell, 1987; Caning, Hanser, Shade, & Boyce, 1993), it may suggest that caregivers are not always aware of the degree of their child's distress. Of equal concern was that the prevalence of overanxious symptoms almost doubled from Time 1 to Time 3 (7%-13%). While these numbers remain relatively low, it appears that with the natural course of the disease and the disruption it brings in its stead, the lives of HIV-infected children will become cumulatively more stressful. As a result, the increase in reported ADHD symptoms, anxiety, and depression may well continue to increase over time and need to be assessed by both child and caregiver report on a routine basis.

In general, the data presented here support and underscore the resilience reported in the Bose (1994) study. That is, despite the demands of a chronic illness, frequent hospital visits, and daily medication, children's psychological functioning remained relatively stable over a two-year period of time. Again, this does not mean that these children will automatically continue to adapt well when confronted with other developmental and life stressors. These children had only been diagnosed an average of 64.58 months. As the crisis of learning of the diagnosis passes, longer-term issues such as the child's concerns about secrecy, disclosure, adolescent sexuality, cumulative losses, and the reality of the seriousness of their illness will evoke new psychological challenges. Clearly, the adaptation of children living with HIV throughout their school-age years and into adolescence requires further (longitudinal) investigation.

Limitations and Implications for Future Research

The generalizability of the present findings is limited by our sample, which over-represented physically and economically resourceful families who were able to involve their child in clinical trials at the NIH. While this allowed us to evaluate the impact of HIV on children's psychological distress apart from the powerful confounding psycholgical risk factors associated with economic deprivation, this study should be replicated in a community/urban setting in order to better represent the population of children living with HIV in the U.S. This study did not ask the children about their specific knowledge of the implications of their disease, such as whether or not they thought that they were going to die from it. Future research would benefit from an exploration of the relationship between psychological distress symptoms and the extent to which the child understands the physical consequences and potential terminal nature of his/her illness. In addition, future studies should explore the impact of the child's temperament, HIV-related illnesses, social and scholastic competence and the additive effect of the multiple losses experienced by many of these children, on their psychological well-being. The latter is especially important when considering that many of these children will experience the deaths of their mothers, fathers, and/or siblings and therefore may require a new care giver at some point during their childhood (Caldwell et al., 1992).

CONCLUSIONS

The results of the study must be considered preliminary findings that warrant further investigation. However, they do have direct applicability for pediatric health care professionals as well as for research investigators. While the prevalence of psychological distress symptoms was not alarmingly high, the increasing nature of both anxiety and depression in our sample suggests that these children may be at risk for psychiatric morbidity. However, both clinicians and investigators who are interested in identifying children who are at risk for psychological difficulties need to begin looking beyond "living with HIV." Often times, these children demonstrate an enormous amount of resilience in coping with the health-related aspects of their lives, only to demonstrate difficulty in school, with peer relationships, and later, in the transition from childhood to adolescence. It is important to better understand how the impact of living with HIV influences normal developmental phenomena such as the increasing influence of peers during the adolescence years. Research has also demonstrated that psychosocial outcomes for chronically ill children are influenced by the psychological functioning of their families. This study supported that finding as family conflict was positively correlated with parental depression, parental anxiety and a report of the child's total behavior problems. Clinicians and researchers alike would be wise to direct their attention toward the functioning of the entire family, those living with HIV/AIDS, and those within the family that are affected by it. The long-term emotional impact on both the infected and surviving members of the family is only beginning to be understood. Public health planners and policy makers must not lose sight of AIDS as a family problem.

Clearly, with the rapid treatment advances within the HIV epidemic, children are living well beyond what had originally been projected. With lengthened survival comes many psychosocial challenges. In addition to the physiological and behavioral changes that will occur in this population, health care providers need to be familiar with issues pertaining to confidentiality, autonomy, medication needs, community resources, legal considerations, sexual identity, and self-esteem (Riddel & Moon, 1996). It is essential that we pay equal attention to the mental health needs of these children as we do their complex medical management. With comprehensive assessment, intervention and support, these children may well be our health care providers of tomorrow.

REFERENCES

Achenbach, T.M. (1991). *Manual for the Child Behavior Checklist /4-18 and 1991 Profile*. Burlington, VT: University of Vermont Department of Psychiatry.

Achenbach, T.M., McConaughy, S.H., & Howell, L.T. (1987). Child/adolescent behavioral and emotional problems: Implications of cross-informant correlations for situational specificity. *Psychological Bulletin, 10*, 213-232.

Austin, J.K. & Huberty T.J. (1993). Development of the child attitude towards illness scale. *Journal of Pediatric Psychology, 18*, 467-480.

Barkley, R.A. (1990). Associated problems, subtyping, and etiologies. In R. A. Barkley (Ed.), *Attention deficit hyperactivity disorder: A handbook for diagnosis and treatments* (pp. 77-105). New York: Guilford Press.

Beck, A. T. (1967). *Depression, Clinical, Experimental and Theoretical Aspects*. New York: Harper.

Beck, A.T. & Steer, R.A. (1987). *Beck depression inventory: Manual*. New York: Harcourt Brace Jovanovich, Inc.

Billings, A.G., Moos, R. H., Miller, J.J. III, & Gottlieb, J.E. (1987). Psychosocial adaptation in juvenile rheumatic disease: A controlled evaluation. *Health Psychology, 6.* 343-359.

Blanche, S., Tardiu, M., Duliege, A. et al. (1990). Longitudinal study of 94 symptomatic infants with maternal/fetal HIV infection: Evidence for a bimodal expression of clinical and biological symptoms. *American Journal of the Diseases of Childhood, 144*, 1210-1215.

Blanche, S., Mayaux, M. J., Rouzioux, D., Teglas, J. P., Firtion, G., Monpouxz, F., Ciraru-Vigneron, N., Meier, F., Tricoire, J., & Courpotin, C. (1994). Relation of the course of HIV infection in children to the severity of the disease in their mothers at delivery. *N Engl J Med, 330(5)*, 308-12.

Bose, S., Moss, H., Brouwers, P., Lorion, R., & Pizzo, P.A. (1994). Psychological adjustment of HIV-infected school age children. *Journal of Developmental and Behavioral Pediatrics, 15(3)*, S26-S33.

Breslau, N. (1985). Psychiatric disorder in children with physical disabilities. *Journal of the American Academy of Child Psychiatry, 24*, 87-94.

Brown, L.K., Schultz, J.R., & Gragg, R.A. (1995). HIV-infected adolescents with hemophilia: Adaptation and coping. *Pediatrics, 96(3)*, 459-463.

Bussing, R. & Burket, R.C. (1993). Anxiety and intrafamilial stress in children with hemophilia after the HIV crisis. *Journal of the American Academy of Child and Adolescent Psychiatry, 32*, 562-567.

Butler, K. M., Husson, R. N., Balis, F. M., Brouwers, P., Eddy, J., El-Amin, D., Gress, J., Hawkins, M., Jarosinski, P., Moss, H., Poplack, D., Santacroce, S., Venzon, D., Wiener, L., Wolters, P., & Pizzo, P. A. (1991). Dideoxyinosine in children with symptomatic human immunodeficiency virus infection. *New England Journal of Medicine, 324(3)*, 137-144.

Cadman, D., Boyle, M., Szatmari, P., & Offord, D.R. (1987). Chronic illness, disability, and mental health and social well-being: Findings of the Ontario Child Health Study. *Pediatrics, 79*, 805-813.

Caldwell, M.B., Mascola, L., Smith, W., Thomas, P., Hsu, H-W, Maldonado, Y., Parrott, R., Byers, R., Oxtoby, M., and the Pediatric Spectrum of Disease Clinical

Consortium (1992). Biologic, foster, and adoptive parents: Caregivers of children exposed perinatally to human immunodeficiency virus in the United States. *Pediatrics, 90 (4)*, 603-607.

Caning, E.H., Hanser, S.B., Shade, K.A. & Boyce, W.T. (1993). Maternal distress and discrepancy in reports of psycholpathology in chronically ill children. *Psychosomatics, 34*, 506-511.

Centers for Disease Control and Prevention (1997). *HIV/AIDS Surveillance Report, 9(1)*, 8-18.

Chase, C., Vibbert, M. Pelton, S.I., Coulter, D.L.; & Cabral, H. (1995). Early neurodevelopmental growth in children with vertically transmitted human immunodeficiency virus infection. *Arch Pediatr Adolesc Med, 149(8):*850-5.

Civitello, L.A., Brouwers, P., & Pizzo, P.A. (1993). Neurological and neuropsychological manifestations in 120 children with symptomatic Human Immunodeficiency virus infection. *Annals of Neurology,34*, 481 [Abstract #122].

Daniels, D., Moos, R.H., Billings A. G., & Miller J.J. (1987). Psychosocial risk and resistance factors among children with chronic illness, healthy siblings, and healthy controls. *Journal of Abnormal Child Psychology, 15(2)*, 295-308.

Davis, E., Fennoy, I., Laraque, D., Kanem, N., Brown, G., & Mitchell, J. (1992). Autism and developmental abnormalities in children with perinatal cocaine exposure. *Journal of the National Medical Association, 84*, 315-319.

Drotar, D.D., Agle, D. P., Eckle, C.L., & Thompson, P.A. (1995). Psychological response to HIV positivity in hemophilia. *Pediatrics, 96(6)*, 1062-1069.

Drotar, D.D. (1997). Relating parent and family functioning to the psychological adjustment of children with chronic health conditions: What have we learned? What do we need to know? *Journal of Pediatric Psychology, 22*, 149-165.

Englund, J. A., Baker, C. J., Raskino, C., McKinney, R. E., Lifschitz, M. H., Petrie, B., Fowler, M. G., Connor, J. D., Mendez, H., O'Donnell, K., Wara, D. W., & ACTG 152 Study Team (1996). Clinical and laboratory characteristics of a large cohort of symptomatic, human immunodeficiency virus-infected infants and children. *Pediatric Infectious Disease Journal, 15*, 1025-36.

European Collaborative Study (1990). Neurologic signs in young children with human immunodeficiency virus infection. *Pediatr Infect Dis J, 9*, 402-406.

Grubman, S., Gross, B., Lerner-Weiss, N. et al. (1995). Older children and adolescents living with perinatally acquired human immunodeficiency virus infection. *Pediatrics, 95*, 657-663.

Havens, J. F., Whitaker, A. H., Feldman, J. F., & Ehrhardt, A. A. (1994). Psychiatric morbidity in school-age children with congenital Human Immunodeficiency Virus infection: A pilot study. *Journal of Developmental and Behavioral Pediatrics, 15(Suppl.)*, S18-S25.

Hooper, S. R., Whitt, J. K., Tennison, M., Burchinal, M., Gold, S., & Hall, C. (1993). Behavioral adaptation to Human Immunodeficiency Virus-seropositive status in children and adolescents with hemophilia. *Behavioral Adaptation, 147, 541-545*.

Kovacs, M., Brent, D., Steinberg, T.F., Paulauskas, S., Reid J. (1986). Children's self-reports of psychological adjustment and coping strategies during first year of insulin-dependent diabetes mellitus. *Diabetes Care, 9*, 472-479.

Lavigne, J.V. & Faier-Routman, J. (1993). Correlates of psychological adjustment to pediatric physical disorders: A meta-analytic review and comparison with existing models. *Journal of Developmental and Behaviroal Pediatrics, 14,* 117-123.

Lobato, M.N., Caldwell, M.B., Ng, P., Oxtoby, M.J., & Consortium PSoDC. Encephalopathy in children with perinatally acquired human immunodeficiency virus infection. *Journal of Pediatrics.* 1995; 126:710-715.

Moos, R. H & Moos, B. S. (1993). *Family Environment Scale Manual* (2nd ed.). Palo Alto CA: Consulting Psychologists Press Inc.

Moss, H.A., Wolters, P.L., Brouwers, P., Hendricks, M.L., & Pizzo, P.A. (1996). Impairment of expressive behavior in pediatric HIV-infected patients with evidence of CNS disease. *J Pediatr Psychol., 21(3):*379-400.

Moss, H.A., Brouwers, P., Wolters, P.L., Wiener, L., Hersh, S., & Pizzo, P.A. (1994). The development of a Q-sort behavioral rating procedure for pediatric HIV patients. *J Pediatr Psychol, 19*(1):27-46.

Pless, I B. & Roghmann, K. (1971). Chronic illness and its consequences: Based on three epidemiological surveys. *Journal of Pediatrics, 79,* 351-358.

Pless, I.B. (1984). Clinical assessment: Physical and psychological functioning. *Pediatric Clinics of North America, 31,* 33-45.

Pless, I B., Roghmann, K., & Haggerty, R. J. (1972). Chronic illness, family functioning and psychological adjustment: A model for the allocation of preventive mental health services. *International Journal of Epidemiology, 1(3),* 271-277.

Riddel, J. & Moon, M.W. (1996). Children with HIV becoming adolescents: caring for long-term survivors. *Pediatric Nursing, 22 (3),* 220-227.

Riekert, K., Wiener, L., Battles, H., Drotar, D. (in press). Prediction of psychological distress in school-age children with HIV. *Children's Health Care.*

Rodning, C., Beckwith, L., & Howard, J. (1989). Characteristics of attachment organization and play organization in prenatally drug-exposed toddlers. *Developmental and Psychopathology, 1,* 277-289.

Roelofs, K., Wolters, P., Fernandez-carol, C., van der Vlugt, H., Moss, H., & Brouwers, P. (1996). Impairments in expressive emotional language in children with symptomatic HIV infection: Relation with brain abnormalities and immune function. *Journal of the International Neuropsychological Society, Abstract.*

Ryan, C.M. & Morrow, L.A. (1986). Self-esteem in diabetic adolescents: Relationship between age at onset and gender. *Journal of Consulting and Clinical Psychology, 54,* 730-731.

Schwab-Stone, M., Fallon, T., Briggs, M., & Crowther, B. (1994). Reliability of diagnostic reporting for children aged 6-11 years: A test-retest of the Diagnostic Interview Schedule for Children-Revised. *American Journal of Psychiatry, 151,* 1048-1054.

Shulman, S., Fisch, R. O., Zempel, C. E., Gadish, O., & Chang, P. N. (1991). Children with phenylketonuria: The interface of family and child functioning. *Journal of Developmental and Behavioral Pediatrics, 12,* 315-321.

Spielberger, C. D. (1983). *Manual for the State-Trait Anxiety Inventory (STAI Form Y).* Palo Alto: Consulting Psychologists Press.

Steinhausen, H., Schindler, H., & Stephan, H. (1983). Correlates of psychopathology in sick children: An empirical model. *Journal of American Academy of Child Psychiatry, 22,* 559-564.

Thompson, R. J. Jr., Hodges, K., & Hamlett, K. W. (1990). A matched comparison of adjustment in children with cystic fibrosis and psychiatrically referred and nonreferred children. *Journal of Pediatric Psychology, 15(6),* 745-759.

Thompson, R. J. Jr., Gustafson, K. E., Hamlett, K. W., & Spock, A. (1992). Psychological adjustment of children with cystic fibrosis: The role of child cognitive processes and Maternal adjustment. *Journal of Pediatric Psychology, 17(6),* 741-755.

Thompson, R. J. Jr., Gustafson, K. E. (1996). *Adaptation to chronic childhood illness.* Washington, DC: American Psychological Association.

Thompson, R.J. Jr., Gustafson, K. E., George, L.K., & Spook A. (1994). Change over a 12-month period in the psychologcial adjustment of children and adolescents with cystic fibrosis. *Journal of Pediatric Psycholgoy, 19,* 189-203.

Thompson, R. J. Jr., Gil, K.M., Keith, B.R., Gustafson, K.E. George, L.K., Kinney, T.R. (1994). Psychological adjustment of children with sickle cell disease: Stability and change over a 10 month period. *Journal of Consulting and Clinical Psychology, 62,* 856-860.

Tovo, P. A., DeMartino, M., Gabiano, C., Cappello, N., D'Elia, R., Loy, A., Plebani, A., Zuccotti, G. V., Dallacasa, P., Ferraris, G., et al. (1992). Prognostic factors and survival in children with perinatal HIV infection. *Lancet, 339,* 449-453.

Valla, J. P., Bergeron, L., Bérubé, H., & Gaudet, N. (1994). A structured pictorial questionnaire to assess DSM-III-R based diagnoses in children (6-11 years): Development, validity and reliability. *Journal of Abnormal Child Psychology, 22,* 403-423.

Valla, J. P., Bergeron, L, Bidaut-Russell, M, St-Georges, M, & Gaudet, N. (1997). Reliability of the Dominic-R: A young child mental health questionnaire combining visual and autditory stimuli. *Journal of Child Psychology and Psychiatry, 38(6),* 717-724.

Wallander, J. L., Varni, J. W., Babani, L., Banis, H. T., & Wilcox, K. T. (1988). Children with chronic physical disorders: Maternal reports of their psychological adjustment. *Journal of Pediatric Psychology, 13,* 197-212.

Walker, L.S., Ortiz-Valdes, & Newbrough, J.R. (1989). The role of maternal employment and depression in the psycholgocial adjustment of chronically ill mentally retarded and well children. *Journal of Pediatric Psychology, 14,* 357-370.

Wallander, J.L. & Thompson, R.J., Jr. (1995). Psychosocial adjustment of children with chronic physical conditions. In MD Robers (Ed). *Handbook of Pediatric Psychology* (2nd edition, pp. 124-141). Guilford Press:New York.

Watson D. & Clark L. (1984). Negative affectivity: The disposition to experience aversive emotional states. *Psychological Bulletin, 96,* 465-490.

Wiener, L., Fair, C., & Pizzo, P.A. (1993). Care for the child with HIV infection and AIDS. In A. Armstrong-Dailey & S. Z. Golter (Eds.), *Hospice Care for Children* (pp. 85-104). New York: Oxford University Press.

Wiener, L., Fair, C., Granowsky, R. (in press). Psychosocial aspects of neurologic impairment in children with AIDS. In H. Gendelman, S. Lipton, L. Epstein, & S. Swindells. (Eds.) *Neurological and Neuropsychiatric Manifestations of HIV-1 Infection.* Chapman & Hall Publishers: New York.

Wiener, L. S. & Septimus, A. (1994). Psychosocial support for the child and family. In P. A. Pizzo & C. M. Wilfert (Eds.) *Pediatric AIDS* (2nd ed., pp. 809-828). Baltimore: Williams & Wilkins MD.

The Working Committee on HIV (1996). *Children, and Families. Families in Crisis* New York: Federation of Protestant Welfare Agencies.

A Troubled Present, an Uncertain Future: Well Adolescents in Families with AIDS

Barbara H. Draimin
Jan Hudis
José Segura
Amy Shire

SUMMARY. The needs of well adolescents in families with AIDS have received little attention, despite the growing number of these youth nationwide. This report summarizes the experiences of 59 adolescents aged 10-19 years old and their parents with AIDS. Parents were faced with difficult decisions regarding custody planning and disclosure of serostatus to children: 39% chose not to disclose their illness to their children and 53% had no viable custody plan. Stigma associated with AIDS and social isolation of families intensified the stress families experienced in attempting to cope with these issues. Despite these challenges, families demonstrated tremendous resiliency and effective coping. These interviews demonstrate the importance of outlining methods for professionals to provide: (1) training to help parents decide if, how and when to disclose their serostatus; (2) assistance in planning for the future custody of children; and (3) in-home supportive counseling for

Barbara H. Draimin, DSW, is Executive Director of the Family Center. Jan Hudis, MPH, MPA, is Research Manager of The Family Center. José Segura, MSW, is affiliated with Gay Men's Health Crisis. Amy Shire, MPH, is a consultant.

Address correspondence to: Barbara Draimin, The Family Center, 66 Reade Street, New York, NY 10007.

This work was supported by Grant # 279492 from the National Institute of Mental Health.

[Haworth co-indexing entry note]: "A Troubled Present, an Uncertain Future: Well Adolescents in Families with AIDS." Draimin, Barbara H. et al. Co-published simultaneously in *Journal of HIV/AIDS Prevention & Education for Adolescents & Children* (The Haworth Press, Inc.) Vol. 3, No. 1/2, 1999, pp. 37-50; and: *HIV Affected and Vulnerable Youth: Prevention Issues and Approaches* (ed: Susan Taylor-Brown and Alejandro Garcia) The Haworth Press, Inc., 1999, pp. 37-50. Single or multiple copies of this article are available for a fee from The Haworth Document Delivery Service [1-800-342-9678, 9:00 a.m. - 5:00 p.m. (EST). E-mail address: getinfo@haworthpressinc.com].

© 1999 by The Haworth Press, Inc. All rights reserved.

families, and transitional case management for new guardians. *[Article copies available for a fee from The Haworth Document Delivery Service: 1-800-342-9678. E-mail address: getinfo@haworthpressinc.com]*

KEYWORDS. HIV/AIDS, families, custody planning, permanency planning, disclosure, adolescents, caregiver, social support, stigma, parental death

INTRODUCTION

A mother with AIDS described her greatest concern: "I'm worried sick about my 15-year-old daughter, Maria. Since I told her I have AIDS she doesn't talk to me and she's always in trouble at home and at school. And now, on top of everything else, I can't find anyone who will take care of her if I die." In many families where a parent has AIDS, the precarious future of children is of paramount concern.

The magnitude of the problem of "AIDS orphans" is supported by the results of a 1992 study projecting the numbers of young people surviving the death of a parent with AIDS through the year 2000. Michaels and Levine (1992) estimate that 80,000 children and adolescents nationwide will lose a mother by the turn of this century. Whereas many people imagine that children whose parents live with AIDS are young and infected, over 80% are uninfected and 46% are adolescents (Michaels & Levine, 1992).

Field experiences of social service providers strongly suggest that adolescents in families with HIV/AIDS suffer deep social and psychological trauma (Draimin, Hudis & Segura, 1992). In need of substantial support and guidance, these adolescents are deprived, through the loss of a parent, of crucial relationships and stability at a developmentally vulnerable time. If one adds to these difficulties the non-HIV-related losses and deprivation experienced by many inner-city children on a daily basis, the needs of the adolescents affected by AIDS are numerous and complex.

All families facing the terminal illness of a family member experience profound loss and pain. Families affected by AIDS, however, often experience additional dimensions to their losses; they are affected by severe stigmatization, and frequently have endured multiple AIDS-related and non-AIDS-related losses. In addition, the ill parent is most often a single parent in these families (as, for example, in the

AIDS social service agency described below, where 80% of families are headed by single women). When that parent dies, children are left orphaned, often without other relatives in economically or socially stable enough situations to permanently care for them. These issues make the experience of AIDS among families distinct from other serious illnesses (Wiener & Septimus, 1990).

Little research has been done to date to explore and document the extent of need among these adolescents and the HIV-related issues that must be addressed. Therefore, the purpose of this study was to explore disclosure, custody planning and social support as three key areas requiring attention and resources. The study was conducted by the New York City Division of AIDS Services, which provides case management services to Medicaid-eligible people with AIDS and HIV illness. Most families served by the agency reside in New York City's poorer neighborhoods, facing problems of poverty, inadequate housing, few opportunities for recreation, unsafe streets, and drug use. Forty parents with AIDS and their children were interviewed, using qualitative methods to document the problems and concerns faced by parents and guardians with regard to their adolescent children 10-19 years old. The study explored the needs of these adolescents in order to more clearly define the problem and to develop guidelines for age-appropriate services to help these young people manage the difficult circumstances that confront them.

Having a parent with AIDS is a significant stressor which compounds the already existing struggles faced by these youth, including living with poverty, substance abuse, unstable housing and weak support systems (Levine, 1993). At the same time these youth are assuming increased responsibility at home, they must confront their own risk of infection and cope with the impending death of a parent–a traumatic event which can seriously interfere with social and emotional functioning (Siegel et al., 1990). Youth who are living with a parent with AIDS often cope with stress in ways that put them at greater risk for HIV infection and other negative outcomes. Distressed youth may use drugs as a means of alleviating unpleasant feelings (Rotheram-Borus et al., in press) and coping with frustration or anticipated failure.

The stigma associated with AIDS makes it difficult for adolescents and their families to make use of extended family, friends and the larger community for support (Cates et al., 1990). Withdrawal from interpersonal relationships may also characterize an adolescent's response to loss (Osterweis et al., 1984). Doka (1990) refers to AIDS as a "disenfranchising death" because the fear and panic it generates often results in isolated survivors who do all their grieving alone. Secrecy may be the best coping mechanism available to families with AIDS (Grief & Porembske, 1989). On a practical level, however, secrets can impede understanding, foster isolation, prevent access to services and increase stigma (Abramson, 1990). This makes coping with serious life events an even greater challenge.

Little is known about the short-term effects on the child caused by parental loss through death (Wolkind & Rutter, 1985). Even less is known about the impact of AIDS on family functioning and mental health (Levine, 1990). The literature on maternal loss in childhood indicates that bereaved children are at increased risk for depression (Bifulco et al., 1987), agoraphobia and panic (Tweed et al., 1989), conduct disturbance and suicide (Chiefetz et al., 1989). They are also more likely than their peers to experience academic difficulty, decreased self-esteem and somatic complaints (McKeever, 1983).

METHODOLOGY

Study Population

Profile of Client Families

In December 1991, the Division of AIDS Services was serving 9,200 clients, including 1,500 families. Approximately 38% of these families had at least one adolescent aged 10-19. Ninety-one percent of the agency's families are Latino and African-American, with the majority of households headed by single women who have a past or current history of drug use. The average family has 3.2 children. In 17% of the families there is also an HIV-infected child under the age of 13.

Study Sample

Forty families, including 59 adolescents between the ages of 10 and 19, were interviewed as part of this study. In twenty families the parent with AIDS was alive, receiving agency services, and residing in the household with his or her adolescent children. In the remaining 20 families, the parent with AIDS had died within the previous year and the adolescent was residing with the surviving parent or with a new guardian.

The families were randomly selected from the caseload of a site office in Brooklyn serving the catchment area with the fastest growing caseload of families.

Of the 40 families studied, 58% were Latino and 42% were African-American. White families were not specifically excluded from the study, but the random sampling did not identify any White families.

The vast majority (90%) of study parents were female. Of those women, 28 were single mothers and eight had male partners who also lived in the household. In none of those eight cases was the male partner also the father of any of the children, nor was he named in the custody plan.

Client Recruitment, Engagement and Interviewing

Protecting the client's confidentiality and maintaining respect for each family's decision on how to handle disclosure of the parent's HIV status to the children were of the highest priority and greatly influenced the study's recruitment strategy and interviewing process. The researchers avoided use of the terms "AIDS" and "HIV," either spoken or in writing, unless the study participant used them. At first contact, researchers identified themselves only as coming from the agency providing entitlements. Any questions asked by teenagers regarding their parent's illness were acknowledged as important but as requiring a response from the parent.

Assessments

Qualitative, face-to-face interviews were conducted with the teens, as well as the youth's parent or guardian. Each interview began with the creation of a genogram to delineate family structure (McGoldrick & Gerson, 1985). Adolescents and their parent or guardian were interviewed separately, using a guided questionnaire with a combination of open and closed responses developed by the research team. Questions addressed such issues as family members' losses; their support systems; adolescents' feelings toward and performance in school; adolescents' responsibilities at home; and parental HIV disclosure and custody planning. Interviews averaged three hours and were conducted in the family's home late in the afternoon or on weekends.

FINDINGS AND DISCUSSION

The many findings of this study have been grouped under three major headings: disclosure, custody planning and social support. These three domains frame our discussion of the problems and suggest ways in which these issues might be addressed through new program development and professional training.

Disclosure

Interviews with parents and new guardians documented significant difficulties with disclosure, both within and outside the family unit. Some of the parents interviewed and many of those who had died had chosen not to inform all or some of their children of their HIV status. Thirty-nine percent of youth interviewed did not know that the parent had AIDS. Many parents indicated that their decision not to inform was based on a desire to protect the child. Often they felt that a child, even an adolescent, was too young or immature to understand or deal with the information. Many parents said they simply did not wish to burden their children with the knowledge that they were very sick and probably going to die. Others said that they feared the youth would inadvertently reveal the parent's HIV status to others, potentially resulting in discrimination toward the entire family. In cases where the parent had not informed the child, the new guardian was left to wrestle with this issue after the parent's death.

Informing their children about their HIV diagnosis was one of the most difficult tasks these parents faced during the course of their illness. For instance, the revelation of a parent's HIV status often involved other stigma-ridden secondary disclosures such as acknowledgment of substance abuse or "unsanctioned" sexual activity.

The interviews illuminated the importance of planned, rather than inadvertent or casual, disclosure. In some cases, parents felt that disclosing their HIV diagnosis to their children had been a huge mistake. One mother who had disclosed to her 18-, 15-, and 7-year-old children on the advice of her hospital social worker compared the experience to "dropping a bomb with no plan for the clean-up." In this family and others, the adolescent children most frequently coped with a parent's illness through denial, refusing to discuss matters such as future custody arrangements, or anticipatory grief for their parent. In families where the children had learned that the parent had AIDS from gossip in the neighborhood, or through the inadvertent disclosure of the parent's illness by a healthcare provider, there was often tremendous anger and resentment toward the parent on the part of the adolescent.

Very few families had chosen to reveal their HIV status outside the family. Of the 61% of adolescents interviewed who knew of their parent's HIV status, none had shared that information with their best friend. Thus the demands of keeping secrets often resulted in the youth being socially isolated. The consequences of outside disclosure could often be severe: in cases where neighbors and others in the community suspected that a family member might have HIV, these families were often subjected to harassment, threats of violence, and the need to relocate to neighborhoods where their anonymity could be better protected. Relocation to new neighborhoods added to adolescents' experiences of isolation.

Custody Planning

Custody planning represents an important step in parents' acknowledgment of their illness and in the ability to plan for their children's future. Custody planning for minor children is a crucial task, often the most painful one a parent must face. Planning for children's futures depends upon the ill person's awareness and acknowledgment of their illness and a willingness to deal with that reality. This study found that even when plans for the children had been set, formalized, legal custody arrangements were rarely made. In 53% of the families in which the parent with AIDS was alive, there was no viable custody plan for the adolescent children. For others, the issue had not been dealt with at all or was addressed only when a health crisis compelled action. Custody plans made during such crises were often incomplete or not formalized.

Custody planning for older adolescents was particularly problematic, as their growing independence and "acting out" behavior made relatives reluctant to accept guardianship responsibility. It was not unusual in these families for a relative to agree to be the guardian for the younger children, but refuse responsibility for the adolescent. In several of the families interviewed, older adolescents went to great lengths to try to keep all of their siblings together in one household. In some cases, this pitted older adolescents against adult family members who might have wished to take custody of the younger children, but who had no interest in accepting the older adolescent into their home.

With other families, legalization of custodial arrangements was complicated when children had different fathers, sometimes resulting in sibling separation at the time of the mother's death. Custody plans often placed children with guardians in fragile health and without the financial and housing resources for their expanded household.

Often, the options for custody depended upon such fundamental criteria as who had room. Biological ties were often not the only important factor in parental custody decisions, and in many cases, uncertainty in custody arrangement was a direct result of a poverty of resources. For families where the cultural expectation is that extended family will automatically take in a parentless child, the entire concept of formal custody may be perceived as alien or insulting.

Stigma, Social Support and Family Coping

The families in this study had experienced a great deal of loss in their lives even prior to any HIV illness, and often their sources of emotional support during crises were undependable. In addition, a tremendous level of AIDS-associated stigma surrounded these families, engendering secretiveness and separation from other family members and community resources (schools, churches, neighbors) when openness and support seemed most desired and needed. This combination of tremendous loss, inconsistency of emotional support, and AIDS-associated stigma often resulted in profound social isolation. Many of the adolescents were acting out their most disturbing emotions. Their behavior confused and distracted adults, keeping parents, teachers, and case managers so preoccupied with the surface behaviors that they were unable to address the underlying emotional issues involved.

Multiple losses, siblings with different fathers and parental drug use resulting in household instability before AIDS in the family all contributed to the complexity of the families interviewed. Multiple losses compounded the isolation of families, strained already fragile coping skills and reduced the number of family members available to take custody of surviving children. Interviews revealed that on average, adolescents had experienced four major losses (e.g., death, divorce, incarceration of significant other, drug addiction) in the previous two years and that over 80% had experienced at least one loss.

Siblings with different fathers added another level of complexity to family life and mothers' plans for their children's future. Fathers often had differing levels of involvement with their children, creating inequalities in the outside resources available to siblings living in the same household. Following the death of the mother, a child with an involved father often went to live in the father's household or in the household of a paternal relative. Those children without an involved father usually went to live with a maternal relative, usually a grandmother or an aunt.

Parental substance use was a characteristic of many of the families interviewed, contributing to frequent changes in household location and composition and often connected with a history of inadequate parenting. Many of the adolescents in these families had at some time in their lives been removed by the city's child welfare agency from the parental household or had been voluntarily placed by the mother in the care of a responsible family member.

The families had extraordinary reserves of strength. Single mothers coping with their own terminal illness displayed enormous care and compassion for their children, while extended family members often took over much of the day-to-day parenting. With AIDS in some communities taking the lives of an entire generation of young parents, it was not unusual to interview a grandmother or an aunt caring for more than one daughter's or sister's children. Indeed, mothers and sisters of the women with AIDS, in particular, were often the "glue" holding these families together.

Adherence to a belief in God was clearly integral to many families' abilities to cope with painful situations. Ironically, however, though many families with AIDS found strength through church affiliations, none disclosed their own HIV status to other congregation members. One couple interviewed visited people with AIDS in hospitals as part of a church-sponsored activity, while continuing to keep their own illness a secret.

Assessment of adolescent social support networks revealed that 38% of the adolescents had no best friend. For these youth, classmates and neighbors were "associates" whom they did not trust enough to consider a true friend. Many adolescents' best friend was a sibling, cousin or other age mate already closely connected with the family. In terms of professional therapeutic assistance, forty-three percent of youth had some form of counseling and 76% had found it satisfactory, though few were in counseling at the time of the interviews. Of those 43%, the vast majority had obtained counseling through the school system.

Thirty-four percent of adolescents interviewed were behaving in problematic ways at home, 73% had problems in school and 58% had experienced a decrease in school grades associated with the illness of the parent. Twenty-five percent of the adolescent boys had had recent experience with law enforcement, including three who had been jailed.

Sixteen of the older adolescents interviewed filled out a self-report questionnaire on their sexual activity and drug use and that of their family and friends. Of the 16 youth who reported, nine had had sexual intercourse at least once. Four out of the five girls had been pregnant at least once and one of the four boys reported that he had fathered a child. In terms of drug use, three youth reported that they used marijuana, one youth reported crack use by family members and two youth reported use of other illicit drugs by family or friends. These data indicate that the adolescents interviewed are exposed to and often engage in high-risk activity. Of particular concern is the large number of pregnancies, indicating a high degree of unprotected sex.

At the close of their interviews, adolescent study participants were asked what they would ask for if they were granted three wishes. Their responses (see Figure 1) indicate the salience of their parent's illness in their lives, as well as their concern about the stability of their family's living situation.

IMPLICATIONS FOR SOCIAL WORK PRACTICE

Counseling

While many of the families interviewed showed remarkable reserves of strength and demonstrated an unusual ability to rally in the

FIGURE 1

If you could have three wishes in the world, what would they be?

TO HAVE MY MOTHER ALIVE, TO HAVE A MOTHER AND FATHER, AND TO LIVE IN A WORLD WHERE THERE WERE NO DRUGS, LYING OR STEALING.

TO CURE MY MOM, TO DO WELL IN SCHOOL, AND FOR THE WORLD TO BE GOOD.

TO HAVE A DRUG-FREE COUNTRY, TO LIVE WHERE NO ONE WOULD EVER DIE AND TO LIVE WITH MY AUNT SUSAN.

face of profound difficulties, progressive illness inevitably strained their coping skills. The unique nature of the AIDS-related losses, coupled with the pattern of shame, secrecy, and isolation surrounding them, lend urgency to the need for increased counseling services for adolescents and other family members affected by AIDS. Families interviewed indicated they could benefit greatly from supportive counseling, including bereavement counseling and support groups for adolescents and new guardians. Many families were willing to consider counseling but experienced multiple barriers to receiving such services, including fear of the mental health system, ethnic and language barriers, and long waiting lists for services at community mental health centers. In addition, some custodial families may feel threatened by the stigma associated with seeking counseling, fearing that if they bring their child for help, a child protective agency may interpret this as evidence of severe trouble at home and interfere with the custody arrangement.

Sensitivity both to the need for privacy and to some families' reluctance to deal with the traditional structure of office visits requires the flexibility to meet with families in their homes or other settings of their choice. Therefore, short-term, in-home, culturally appropriate counseling services to both adults and youth in families experiencing AIDS-related losses should be developed. Other service models deserving further investigation include transitional case management services for new guardians and group interventions in which families can learn from and support one another. Telephone and in-person support groups can provide safe forums for sharing information, feelings and coping strategies. Buddy programs for non-infected family members also warrant investigation. Also needed are structured, time-limited group programs that bring infected parents together to build the skills they need for improving communication with their children and for formulating and implementing viable custody plans for all of their children.

Advocacy

The youth interviewed in this study needed advocates in the school and court systems. This is particularly true of youth in families plagued by drug use, illness and unstable living situations, who were unlikely to have family members willing or able to advocate for them. In addition, youth need programs that recognize their needs, including flexible school schedules allowing them to be home with a sick parent when necessary. This is especially vital for older teens who must often assume a great deal of responsibility in the home during the parent's illness.

Professional Training

In addition to the development of specific types of counseling and support services, this assessment of service needs confirmed a need for community-based services with youth providers who are sensitive to the special needs of families with HIV. Training which addresses the complex issues of disclosure, custody planning, mental health issues, social support, legal service concerns, and advocacy is paramount for all professionals working with families with HIV/AIDS.

Training for professionals on custody planning is a growing, unmet need. Custody planning demands facility in personal problem-solving and a sophisticated understanding of legal and entitlement issues. Professionals need to understand all three dimensions before they can assist mothers formulating custody plans for their children.

The perspective shared by many social service professionals is that being open about one's illness is generally emotionally healthier, and that, particularly in terms of its effects on children, having family secrets tends to backfire and cause confusion and resentment. In serving parents with AIDS, there is a professional temptation to try to speed the process of disclosure and custody planning as a response to the fear that the impending death of the parent will leave families in chaos. With fifty percent of the parents studied dying without a custody plan, this fear is not unfounded.

Making and implementing decisions about disclosure and custody planning are among the most difficult tasks faced by parents with AIDS. Appreciation is required for the process parents go through in making these decisions and respect for the complex issues they confront. Disclosure is sometimes viewed simplistically as a "tell-everything-or-tell-nothing" event. Both clients and professionals assume that disclosure of the client's illness must necessarily incorporate disclosure of HIV as well. However, disclosure of HIV may occur gradually along a continuum of partial disclosures. For example, an HIV-positive mother might reveal her situation first by explaining that she is ill, later discussing the seriousness of the illness, and still later speaking about its terminal nature. This may all have taken place without disclosing HIV. Sensitivity to the differing levels of disclosure allows those who would like to remain private about HIV to get on with the task of planning for their children's futures.

Sensitivity on the part of mental health providers toward following the family's pace in making decisions regarding disclosure is critical. Optimally, disclosure of HIV/AIDS takes place in a supportive atmosphere where the parent feels capable of responding appropriately to his or her children's reactions or has assistance in doing so. Careful assessment of the family's communication skills must be done before making the disclosure option part of the therapeutic process.

The social worker's goal is to support family resiliency by developing programs that will assist parents, children, and new guardians in leading healthy, constructive lives in the face of enormous loss.

REFERENCES

Abramson, M. (1990). Keeping secrets: Social workers and AIDS. *Social Work, 35*(2), 169-173.

Bifulco, A.T., Brown, G.W., & Harris, T.O. (1987). Childhood loss of parent, lack of adequate parental care and adult depression. *Journal of Affective Discord, 12*(2), 115-128.

Cates, J.A., Graham, L.L., Boeglin, D., & Tielker, S. (1990). The effect of AIDS on the family system. *Families in Society, 71*(4), 195-201.

Cheifetz, P.N., Stavrakakis, G., and Lester, E.P. (1989). Studies of the affective state in bereaved children. *Canadian Journal of Psychiatry, 34*(7), 688-692.

Doka, K.J. (1990). Grief education: Educating about death for life. In G. Anderson (Ed.), *Courage to care: Responding to the Crisis of children with AIDS*. Washington, DC: Child Welfare League.

Draimin, B.H., Hudis, J., Segura, J. (1991). *The Mental Health Needs of Well Adolescents in Families with AIDS*. New York City Human Resources Administration Division of AIDS Services, New York, New York.

Grief, G. and Porembski, E. (1989). Implications for therapy with significant others of persons with AIDS. *Journal of Gay and Lesbian Psychotherapy, 1*, 79-86.

Levine, C. (1990). AIDS and changing concepts of family. *The Milbank Quarterly, 68*(1), 33-58.

Levine, C. (1993). Introduction. In Levine, C., ed. *A Death in the Family: Orphans of the HIV Epidemic*. p. xii. New York, NY: The United Hospital Fund.

McGoldrick, M.,& Gerson, R. (1985). *Genograms and Family Assessment*. New York, NY: W.W. Norton.

McKeever. P. (1983). Siblings of chronically ill children: A literature review with implications for research and practice. *American Journal of Orthopsychiatry, 53*(2), 209-217.

Michaels, D., & Levine, C. (1992). Estimates of the number of motherless youth orphaned by AIDS in the United States. *Journal of the American Medical Association, 268* (24), 3456-3461.

Osterweis, M., Solomon, F. & Green, M. (Eds.) (1984). *Be-reavement: Reactions, consequences and care.* Washington, DC: National Academy Press.

Rotheram-Borus, M., Rosario, M. & Koopman, C. (In press). Minority youth at risk: Gay males and runaways. In S. Gore & M.E. Coltten (Eds.), *Adolescent, Stress and Coping.* Hawthorne, New York: Aldine de Gruyter.

Siegel, K., Mesagno, F., & Christ, G. (1990). A prevention program for bereaved children. *American Journal of Orthopsychiatry 60*, (2), 168-175.

Tweed, J.L., Schoenbach, V.J., George, L.K., and Blazer, D.G. (1989). The effects of childhood parental death and divorce on six-month history of anxiety disorders. *British Journal of Psychiatry, 154*, 823-828.

Wiener, L., & Septimus, A. (1990). Psychological consideration and support for the child and family. In P. Pizzo (ed.), *Pediatric AIDS: The challenge of HIV infection in infants, children, and adolescents.* pp. 577-594. New York, NY: William and Wilkins.

Wolkind, S., & Rutter, M. (1985). Separation loss and family relationships. In Rutter and Hersov (Eds.), *Child and adolescent psychiatry: Modern approaches.* London, England: Blackwell Scientific Publishers.

The Impact
of Targeted Prevention Programs
for Adolescents at High Risk
for HIV Transmission

Kelly Ward
Judith Waters

SUMMARY. Although most cases of HIV infection have been detected in men and women in their twenties and thirties, due to the long incubation period, it is assumed that they acquired the virus during adolescence. Despite the fact that in most geographic areas of the country, HIV transmission has involved homosexual contact, in our inner cities, the spread of Acquired Immunodeficiency Syndrome (AIDS) has primarily been through the sharing of contaminated injection drug paraphernalia and sexual contact with infected users, again during the teenage years. It is clear that early prevention programs which incorporate drug use issues are essential. Adolescent clients, however, present very difficult barriers for prevention programs since they frequently engage

Kelly Ward, LCSW, CADC, is Instructor, Monmouth University, Social Work Department.

Judith Waters, PhD, is Professor of Psychology and Director of the Masters Program in Addictions Counseling at Fairleigh Dickinson University.

Address correspondence to Kelly Ward, Social Work Department, Monmouth University, Cedar Ave., West Long Branch, NJ 07764.

The writers would like to extend their appreciation to the staff and administrators of Integrity Inc., Newark, New Jersey, where the data were collected.

This research was supported by a Center for Disease Control and Prevention Grant # U65/CCU201540-02.

[Haworth co-indexing entry note]: "The Impact of Targeted Prevention Programs for Adolescents at High Risk for HIV Transmission." Ward, Kelly, and Judith Waters. Co-published simultaneously in *Journal of HIV/AIDS Prevention & Education for Adolescents & Children* (The Haworth Press, Inc.) Vol. 3, No. 1/2, 1999, pp. 51-77; and: *HIV Affected and Vulnerable Youth: Prevention Issues and Approaches* (ed: Susan Taylor-Brown and Alejandro Garcia) The Haworth Press, Inc., 1999, pp. 51-77. Single or multiple copies of this article are available for a fee from The Haworth Document Delivery Service [1-800-342-9678, 9:00 a.m. - 5:00 p.m. (EST). E-mail address: getinfo@haworthpressinc.com].

© 1999 by The Haworth Press, Inc. All rights reserved.

in magical thinking, have poor impulse control, either believe they are invincible or suffer from low self-esteem, in addition to abusing drugs. The Centers for Disease Control and Prevention funded a prevention program in Newark, New Jersey, to target particularly challenging groups: males in the Essex County Youth Detention Center, pregnant teenagers, and welfare recipients (both adults and adolescents). Unfortunately, the research results indicate that despite a high level of knowledge about HIV, in all groups, several dangerous myths still exist. Furthermore, since many of these youth and adults continue to deny their high-risk status, they are relatively unmotivated to develop self-protective lifestyles and safer sexual practices. Suggestions for improved prevention programs are discussed. *[Article copies available for a fee from The Haworth Document Delivery Service: 1-800-342-9678. E-mail address: getinfo@ haworthpressinc.com]*

KEYWORDS. Adolescents, AIDS, HIV prevention

THE NATURE OF THE PROBLEM

In October of 1997, a shocked public was informed about the alleged behavior of Nushawn Williams, a young man of 20 who had engaged in unprotected sex with at least 28 women (a significant number of whom were teenagers), even after he learned that he was seropositive. Many of his partners have now acquired the AIDS virus and, in turn, have probably infected their other partners. According to a *New York Times* article (Sexton, 1997), in addition to drugs and coercion, Nushawn Williams also used his charm and his image of being a "big city gangster" to influence the women, some as young as 13 years of age. He would cook for them or take them shopping for gifts. He is also said to have protected at least one of his partners from threats by other men. When Mr. Williams's behavior was uncovered, he was already being held at the Rikers Island correctional facility in New York City on unrelated rape charges involving a 13-year-old girl and could eventually face at least 10 additional assault charges (Reuters, 1997). He informed authorities that, in addition to the 28 women in Chautauqua County in western New York State, he had sexual contact with from 50 to 75 women in New York City. New York City officials say that at least 11 new HIV cases can be traced to Mr. Williams. The newspaper, radio, and television accounts of Mr. Williams's coercion or seduction (using the promise of drugs) of these women tend to focus on *his* family

background and his personal history of violent and drug-related activities. However, the real emphasis should be on why there were many
cooperative (or semi-cooperative) women who were willing to risk
their lives for an unprotected sexual encounter with Mr. Williams. Were
they ignorant of the facts of HIV transmission? Were they in denial of
the very real dangers? Was Mr. Williams so attractive that they lost the
ability to control their impulses?

The answer for at least some of these women involves the lure of
drugs. The answers for others may have included the threat of violence
(Mr. Williams has a record of being a violent man), the desire to
engage in dangerous behaviors, and/or simply that lack of impulse
control. As a society, we must ask ourselves why we have done such a
poor job of preparing the youth of America to take care of themselves
and to assume responsibility for the future of this nation.

The Centers for Disease Control and Prevention (CDC) Division of
STD Prevention report (June, 1995) that, as compared with older
adults, adolescents in the ten- to 19-year-old age group and young
adults 20 to 24 years old are at higher risk for contracting all categories of sexually transmitted diseases (STDs). There are several reasons
postulated for their vulnerability. For example, young people are more
apt to be involved in several relationships (either sequentially or con-
currently) rather than in a monogamous long-term relationship. They
are likely to engage in unprotected sex and to be involved with partners who have themselves followed the same high-risk behavioral
patterns. Since, in recent years, there is a growing gap between the age
of first sexual contact and the age of marriage (marriage in itself does
not guarantee either monogamy or safety), the vulnerable period of
premarital sex and the risk of STDs or unwanted pregnancy has increased considerably (Waters, Roberts, & Morgan, 1997). In addition,
especially in neighborhoods where the population is impoverished,
there are a number of barriers to the utilization of prevention services
that contribute to the adolescents' risk level including "inability to
pay, lack of transportation, discomfort with facilities and services
designed for adults, and concerns with confidentiality" (Division of
STD Prevention 1995, p. 2). A number of authors have also related
economic issues (Wilson, 1996), drugs (Califano, 1995; Robertson &
Waters, 1994), racial marginalization (Martell & Schinke, 1991), community disorganization (Sampson, Raudenbush, & Earls, 1997) to the
increased incidence of a broad spectrum of mental and physical disor-

ders. Many adolescents (both male and female) in our decaying inner cities also engage in the exchange of sex for money or drugs which places them in the most vulnerable risk category.

Vulnerability to HIV infection is definitely related to geographic area. In the most recent report (December 31, 1997), the CDC lists the ten states or territories with the highest count of AIDS cases. New York leads the way (120,102) followed by California (104,756), Florida (64,906), Texas (44,501), and New Jersey (36,110) (where the authors work and live). Some cities actually have more AIDS cases than entire states. New York City has over 100,000 cases (101,670) which outranks the whole state of Florida and is close to the state of California. New York City is followed by Los Angeles (37,083). Newark, which once would have ranked sixth in a list of states, is now 11th in the listed cities (14,553). The change in its status may be explained in a number of ways. First of all, the reporting system in other cities and states may have finally caught up with the actual number of cases in those locations, other areas could have increased more rapidly than Newark, or, what we hope to be the case, the combined efforts of all the prevention programs in Essex County might actually have had an impact on high-risk sexual behavior.

While heterosexual women are now the fastest-growing category of new AIDS cases, adolescent males still constitute the predominant number of patients. According to data cited in Post and Botkin (1995), HIV has presently become the leading cause of death for young men in five states. It now accounts for 29 percent of the mortality rate for those in the 25-44 age category in New York, 28 percent in New Jersey, 24 percent in California and Florida, and 16 percent in Massachusetts. As previously noted, it is probable that many men in this group acquired the disease when they were adolescents.

The rate of HIV transmission is especially high for African American and Latino youth who live in urban environments. These areas are typified by underemployment, poverty, educational decay, drug abuse, and high crime rates, all factors that are hazardous to anyone's physical and social development (Romer, 1995). Of the 34,214 cases of AIDS in New Jersey as of June 30, 1997, most of them were African American males (n = 12,530) followed by white males (7,774), African American females (5,820) and Hispanic males (4,159) (New Jersey HIV/AIDS cases, reported as of June 30, 1997). The largest single category of transmission was injection drug use for African

American males (7,941), which exceeded the total of all categories for white males. African American female injection drug users totaled 3,435, almost twice the total of all white female patients (1,808). Essex County (Newark) accounts for 30 percent (7,253) of the cases followed by Hudson County (Jersey City) with 14 percent (3,391), and Passaic County (Patterson) with 9 percent (2,069).

In a recent national survey of contemporary parental concerns, the results indicate that, in contrast to other categories, low-income urban parents are most anxious about their children's physical safety, vulnerability to both drug abuse and to contracting AIDS, potential for "dropping out" of school early, and the chances that their female children would become pregnant or that their male children would get someone pregnant (Romer, 1995). They are also worried about the lack of services available to counteract negative influences in the community. These are very realistic concerns. The reality is that inner city adolescents are at high risk for all these hazards (Lombardi, Cargill, Stephens, & Gigliotti, 1997). Consequently, the challenge of modifying adolescent sexual behavior cannot be minimized or seen as separate from other risks. As Post and Botkin (1995) have noted, the results of prevention programs designed to promote abstinence or to use contraceptives have been disappointing. One reason may be that the programs were too narrow in focus. It may also be that while few single programs can demonstrate statistically significant rates of risk reduction, the combined influence of the religious institutions, mass media approaches, along with school and community based prevention efforts can actually achieve some of the goals of *Healthy People 2000* (1991) (e.g., risk reduction for HIV transmission). Prevention programs must also address teenage pregnancies (Luker, 1996), crime (Bennett, Dilulio, & Walters, 1997), drug use (Boatler, Knight & Simpson, 1994; Boyer & Ellen, 1994), and other indicators of social decay before we can expect significant change.

The importance of targeting economic problems, educational deficits and crime at the same time as we address high-risk sexual behavior cannot be overemphasized. Even well-designed prevention programs that do not examine the broader range of community needs will be doomed to failure eventually. A recent study highlights the value of total community involvement. In discussing differences in the levels of violence in communities where economic levels have been controlled, Sampson, Raudenbush, and Earls (1997) have developed the concept of "collective efficacy" to explain lower crime rates in neighborhoods where more violence might have been predicted. They define collective efficacy as "social cohesion among neighbors combined with their willingness to intervene on behalf of the common good" (p. 918). Not only is such a phenomenon related to the reduction of violence, but it should also lead to improvements in mental and physical health in the community and hopefully, a reduction in HIV risk factors. For example, in communities with a high level of collective efficacy, the residents are willing to exert social control in situations where children, adolescents, and even other adults are engaging in dysfunctional acts. For teenagers, such interventions involve reporting truancy or stopping them from "hanging out" on street corners. It also means developing alternative methods of utilizing their energy (e.g., the development of challenging after-school programs).

As Sullivan (1996) notes, it is essential to identify and utilize the cofactors that contribute to high-risk behavior for youth when designing prevention programs. Even when the cofactors are incorporated, the process used to enhance behavioral changes is critical. It is clear that education alone is not sufficient. In most (but not all) previous studies, for example, it has already been found that although adolescents have a firm knowledge of the modes of HIV transmission and the risk cofactors (e.g., non-injection drug use that clouds judgment), they still engage in unprotected sexual encounters with high risk partners (Morton, Nelson, Walsh, Zimmerman & Coe, 1996; Katz, Mills, Singh & Best, 1995). Once it was recognized that didactic presentations alone did not lead to behavioral changes, social skills training to resist negative peer pressure, and negotiation, problem solving, and decision making skills began to be incorporated into prevention programs to assist individuals in developing healthy, self-protective lifestyles. Due to the possibility that some participants may still be unaware of all the dangers and may also hold myths that need to be dispelled, a certain amount of knowledge should still be included into any HIV prevention program.

While not all adolescents suffer from the same social problems or exhibit the same personality characteristics, there are a sufficient number who manifest signs of Fetal Alcohol Syndrome or Effect, cognitive deficits, emotional instability, a propensity for risk taking, an unrealistically low or high sense of self-esteem, magical thinking, depression, dependency, and a lack of impulse control (Waters, Roberts, & Morgan, 1997). All too many exhibit symptoms of early child-hood sexual or physical abuse (Farber, Waters, Levine & Hennen, 1995). Such problems require long-term solutions. Among the most serious co-factors is homelessness.

Sullivan (1996) conducted a program to address the needs of run-aways and drug-involved street youth, as well as young prostitutes and their customers. According to Sullivan, the designation of potential participants as high risk was based on the existence of more than one of the following conditions: homelessness, transient, or tenuous hous-ing; involvement with illicit drugs; prostitution in exchange for money, drugs, food, and shelter; and identification as being gay or bisexual. Collectively, these factors constitute a condition of social marginalization that jeopardizes the chances of healthy development (p. 60). According to Sullivan (1996), any or all of the markers of "hard-to reach" populations (e.g., adolescent drug use and prostitu-tion) made initial contact very difficult. He writes that even when initial contact was made, follow-up data collection was challenging to say the least. Consequently, the group of runaway and street youth from whom data were collected constituted a convenience sample (N = 69). Ninety-three percent of the participants were sexually active and were engaged in exchanging sex for money or drugs (fifty-seven percent were willing to accept drugs alone). Sixty percent practiced oral sex without a condom and 53 percent reported anal and/or vaginal sex, also without a condom. Since only 25 percent of the youth were actually registered at school during the term of the project, a school-based program would have missed the majority of the sample. Forty-four percent reported "no fixed addresses or reliable shelter arrange-ments" (p. 62), which, of course, makes them a very vulnerable group for a broad spectrum of high-risk situations. The results of Sullivan's data collection indicated that 13 percent could not answer the basic questions about HIV transmission. When queried about sources of infection, 25 percent made at least one mistake. As previously found, however, even when there was accurate knowledge, it did not general-ize to behavioral risk reduction. For example, only 20 percent reported that they consistently used condoms.

Post and Botkin (1995) express serious concern about the content of some prevention programs. They cite knowledge about the use of condoms. According to the authors, the use of condoms, even with spermicide, does not guarantee complete safety from HIV transmission. Not all youth know or seem to remember that fact. Moreover, proper usage is not always employed. Unfortunately, for sexually active teenagers, complete abstinence or a monogamous relationship with a mutually faithful, non-injection-drug-using, uninfected partner remains the only completely safe alternative. Not an easy goal to achieve in cities such as Newark.

Since adolescents and adults in our society seem to treat transient sexual encounters as a recreational activity, a significant proportion of the population will continue to risk unplanned pregnancies, sexually transmitted diseases, and even death for a casual affair or the mere chance of a long-term relationship. The problem is further complicated by the fact that many youth have a history of early physical intimacy sometimes in the form of childhood sexual abuse. There are also some important geographic differences that influence HIV transmission rates (Post & Botkin, 1995). In many regions in this country, the age of first intimacy is 12, although the national average is actually about 16 years of age. One would be naive to expect controlled behavior at such early ages, especially if the first contact is some form of incest.

While we have not yet discussed peer pressure in adolescents, it is clearly a factor to be considered. For example, the theory of reasoned action (Greene, Hale, & Rubino, 1997) states that what others think about a behavior will influence the performance of that behavior, especially if the individual thinks it is important to conform to these norms. When the person's own attitudes and the subjective norms of his or her peers coincide, we face a very formidable set of predisposing factors.

While drug abuse is an important factor, the use of so-called "hard drugs" is not solely responsible for high-risk sexual behavior. Mark Ebenhoch, an openly gay man, being interviewed by Green (1996) in a *New York Times Magazine* article said, "Alcohol is a tool to free yourself to destroy yourself if you already want to. And no poster is going to solve that" (p. 43). Ebenhoch noted there is also a strong tendency to rationalize unsafe behavior by discounting the risk involved, by saying to oneself, "This is okay now because . . ." (the reader may substitute any excuse available). Ebenhoch continues, "Sometimes you'd go home with somebody you might not want because of loneliness, and in that position I sure wouldn't mention safe sex. I'd always wait for them to say something about it . . . But no one did" (p. 40). Loneliness is a factor that should not be minimized. It has been suggested that loneliness is the most serious psychological problem in the United States today.

Prevention professionals are distressed by the fact that, while initially successful, the prevention campaign designed by the gay community eventually failed. Green (1996) points out that the difficulties in motivating people to change private behavior either for their own good or for the good of the public have remained a chronic problem (p. 40). For example, programs designed to reduce drug use by adolescents and teenage pregnancies have not led to noticeable reductions in those targeted behaviors (Roberts & Waters, 1998). Of course, one could reasonably argue that the situation would be even worse without such campaigns. Green (1996) attributes the failure of prevention efforts to the focus on abstinence alone, the "Just Say No" approach of the Reagan Presidency. It is very difficult for the average person to withdraw or abstain from sexual activity, even when one feels guilty about the way that others may be endangered. Moreover, some people, both teenagers and adults, think that taking precautions against AIDS is a waste of time and effort since they are convinced that they will acquire the disease sooner or later despite their efforts. Others, of course, engage in magical thinking, feeling themselves to be immortal.

The issues of fidelity, exclusivity, trust, and romance are salient as well. If one partner has had a sexual encounter outside of a supposedly monogamous relationship, he or she should warn the other person. Since the consequences of disclosure can be abandonment, we should not expect such altruistic behavior often. The romance factor also plays a significant role in unprotected sex. Teenagers and even adults dream of encounters that are instinctive, spontaneous, and almost like a scene from a movie or a novel; no one wants to shatter the romantic illusion of the moment. Romantic encounters, especially for adolescents, usually occur quickly leaving little time or inclination for negotiation, preparation, or informed refusal.

Green (1996) discusses the plight of lonely adolescent women as an analogy to the challenge of reducing high-risk sex in the gay community: "Strangely, I'm reminded of the dilemma of poor teenagers for whom sex and even pregnancy may be a way of repairing, if only temporarily, a damaged sense of self-esteem. No wonder campaigns aimed at holding such girls to a vow of chastity, or that simply throwing birth control at them has so little chance of working" (p. 44).

In Green's article, Mark Ebenhoch says, "I don't think I have it now [AIDS], but I probably will eventually. And if I do, it'll be from hooking up with the wrong person, a lonely person, a person who doesn't have the feeling he has any reason to care–someone like me' (p. 44).

Prevention professionals have hoped that it would be possible to teach both adolescents and adults to utilize the model of rational self-interest in making important life decisions. In other words, empower teenagers to ask what the costs and what the rewards are for any behavior. The question is what price will people, especially adolescents, pay for the promise of love and for the possibility of a long-term relationship. According to Green, the problem isn't sex but love. The need for love and "belongingness" have long been recognized as powerful forces. Green further suggests that,

> Instead of promoting vows of chastity, pregnancy prevention programs might ask a girl to envision the kind of life she wants before weighing how a baby could enhance or ruin it. What all such programs would rely on is candor. Complete information, delivered in plain language, respectful of individual values which seems obvious until you realize it is rarely done. And the bitterest pill in prevention today is that the programs already exist. Largely unfinanced or ignored, they sit even now in bookcases and file drawers, waiting for political winds to shift while the epidemic rages. (p. 85)

THE COMPONENTS OF GOOD PREVENTION PROGRAMS

As we noted previously, prevention professionals engaged in trying to modify all sorts of high-risk behaviors in adolescents (e.g., criminal activity and drug and alcohol use), but most especially unprotected sexual encounters, have long since come to the conclusion that educational programs alone are insufficient and that it requires new and creative strategies to influence the attitudes and the behavioral change process (Boyer, Shafer, & Tschann, 1997; Waters, Roberts, & Morgen, 1997; Waters, Morgen, Kuttner, Schmitt, & Schwartz, 1996; Bandura, 1992). Clearly, it is necessary to develop the social skills to withstand negative peer pressures, to be able to negotiate safer sex, and to have the self-esteem and sense of self-efficacy to select, develop, and maintain a healthy, productive, self-protective lifestyle. For example, Boyer, Shafer, and Tschann (1997) review the efficacy of a program implemented in four urban public high schools with a total of 695 students, 513 of whom completed both research instruments (T_1, which was administered one week prior to the beginning of the intervention and T_2, which was administered four weeks after the end of the intervention). The study was a comparison of the relative efficacy of a didactic presentation versus a combination of didactic material plus skills-building strategies. At least 84 percent of the sample (with a mean age of 14.4 and a range of 13-17 years of age) had already experienced vaginal sex, 15 percent had a history of sexually transmitted diseases, 48 percent used alcohol, 18 percent used marijuana and less than 5 percent reported using crack/cocaine, heroin, or other drugs (e.g., Quaaludes). Thirty-nine percent had one to two partners in the previous month with 7 percent having three or more. The mean age of sexual debut was 12.3 years. After controlling for some differences in initial demographic variables, the broad-based intervention process relative to the didactic group had only a small impact on knowledge of sexually transmitted diseases, sexual risk prevention skills and substance use prevention skills but no significant influence on condom use, the number of sexual partners and drug and alcohol use. The authors, however, have concluded that it is premature to assume that the skills-building prevention intervention was unsuccessful. It may be that there will be a "sleeper effect" over time. Moreover, acquiring skills does not necessarily mean that the individual is motivated to move from "preparation for action" to the "action" stage in the Prochaska, DiClemente, and Norcross model of behavioral change (1992).

In the brief publication, *Quick list: Ten steps to a drug-free future* (a component in a drug use prevention campaign targeted toward African American youth), the staff from the Center for Substance Abuse Prevention (CSAP) emphasize the need to nurture, positively reinforce, praise, and give attention to at-risk children and adolescents. They also focus on assuring such youth that they are not alone and that there will be adults such as extended family members, neighbors, and teachers for support, guidance, and love. They further suggest that adults must set a good example and volunteer to help youth within each community. Unfortunately, while there are increasing numbers of volunteers and paid professionals trained to address the challenges of working with today's teenagers, those numbers are clearly insufficient to fill the growing void created by family members who have died from AIDS, drug-related causes, and violence, or who have been incarcerated, or who have abandoned their children for a variety of reasons. The number of self-care ("latch-key") children has grown to the point where after-school programs are quickly filled even in affluent suburbs. In the poverty-stricken inner cities, children have become vagabonds going from house to house for a meal and sometimes even living in old abandoned cars, crack houses, or wherever they can find shelter. Some of them have not been in school for years. Peter Gallione, the Substance Abuse Coordinator for the Campus Program (sponsored by the Juvenile Justice Commission of New Jersey), points out that a system already overburdened with truants cannot keep track of everyone (Personal communication, Peter Gallione, October 29, 1997). It is only when they become involved with the juvenile justice system, including court diversionary programs and other probation-based solutions, that a social worker or probation officer may discover the conditions under which some youth manage to survive.

Although the above-mentioned CSAP publication promotes the value of adult modeling and support, some successful prevention programs try to convince at-risk youth that they, alone, must be responsible for the development of healthy self-protective lifestyles regardless of whether or not they have positive adult influences.

In a four-year longitudinal study of 174 male and female students who were in the ninth grade in 1989, Chubb, Fertan and Ross (1997) found that there was a significant main effect for self-esteem with lower self-esteem for the girls than the boys. This finding reinforces he earlier results of a number of other researchers. The authors point out that low self-esteem has already been related to "low life satisfaction, loneliness, anxiety, restlessness, irritability, and depression" (p. 114). They cite the theory of sociologist C. H. Cooley, entitled "the looking glass self," in which he postulated that self-esteem is a function of how "significant others" view and evaluate us. For young women who have been abused (often both sexually and physically) by the very people responsible for their safety and care, it should come as no surprise that they are vulnerable to the pressures of others in their lives (especially males) and that it is extremely difficult to empower them to develop autonomy and a healthy sense of self. We tend to focus on the sexual abuse of young girls but a study by Farber, Waters,

Levine, and Hennen (1995) discovered that among drug-addicted males, many had been both physically and sexually abused as children. The males were more reluctant to discuss the problem than the females, waiting as long as six months in treatment to raise the issue with their counselors.

Chubb et al. (1997) also studied locus-of-control which logically appears to be related to the concept of self-efficacy with "internals" thinking they are in more control of their lives than "externals." There did not seem to be meaningful differences between gender groups on this variable. Depending on circumstances, both men and women may be "externals." It is our contention, however, that many young women do behave as if they are not capable of functioning effectively without a male in their lives.

In order to address as many of the challenges to HIV prevention as possible in a high-risk community such as Newark, New Jersey, the Centers for Disease Control and Prevention funded a program to reach young participants outside of the school context. While behavioral change is the main goal, the CDC still considers knowledge and attitude change to be critical factors. The grant was given to Integrity House, a drug therapeutic community (T.C.) situated in the center of the drug-dealing world in Newark. The research design was a simple pretest-posttest use of a questionnaire or questionnaires (depending on the program).

In designing prevention and early intervention programs, it is important to sensitize individuals to the dangers of HIV transmission so that they will consider changing their lifestyles and prepare to take realistic action. What should, of course, be avoided is the type of fear-based message that generates denial or a sense of hopelessness. The classic literature on fear-based messages going back over 25 years ago (e.g., Janis & Feshback, 1975) indicates that low levels of fear are not motivating, while high levels are debilitating. The program was designed to elicit the optimum level, a moderate amount of fear which can lead to positive behavioral changes.

CDC provided a technical assistance workshop for all the grantees in the State of New Jersey. Evaluation issues were reviewed and prevention program staff were given guidelines for designing the questionnaires. The CDC was most concerned with assessing whether or not changes in knowledge, attitudes, behavior and beliefs (KABB) have taken place, which virtually mandated the pretest/posttest design.

When this three-year project was first implemented, the focus was on delivery of services to hard-to-reach populations such as youth in detention centers, pregnant teens, and young welfare recipients, all of whom would not be covered in school-based programs. The definition of "hard-to-reach-populations" is not difficult to understand. They are essentially people in the community with whom it is difficult to make initial contact. There is also the implication that further complicated data collection and analysis with this group of participants would be impossible. They were not only hard to reach in the first place, they were extremely difficult to maintain. They were not motivated to remain during the sessions and even if they were physically present (as required in the Youth Detention Center), their minds appeared to be wandering. Clearly, this situation is very frustrating for researchers and evaluators. The alternative is, however, worse and that is not to collect data at all. Please bear with us in this imperfect world and understand that our analysis and interpretations will be somewhat tentative due to the attrition rate. Moreover, one should be very careful in believing that HIV data collected under optimum conditions is literally "carved in stone." For example, myths that we first gathered to develop the questionnaire were no longer held in many cases, others were still supported. Some beliefs about HIV transmission and AIDS were difficult to change. Even when they did, there was no guarantee that behaviors would follow. On the other hand, Newark is no longer ranked sixth in the United States in the number of reported AIDS cases. While it is certainly possible that the best explanation is that other cities and states have caught up, we prefer to believe that the totality of AIDS prevention messages has actually had a positive impact.

NEWARK

When designing any prevention program, the social environment must be taken into account. If Newark were a state it would now rank 11th in the United States in number of reported HIV cases. At one time, it ranked sixth. One baby in 22 is born HIV seropositive at University Hospital in Newark (AIDSline, 1996). In a city such as Newark where unemployment, poor housing, significantly high crime rates, and chemical dependency are typical, and where drop-out rates in some schools are as high as 80 percent, the task is formidable. In Newark, the spread of AIDS is most closely linked to the utilization of intravenous drug paraphernalia or sexual relations with an injection drug user who is already infected and is probably an intravenous drug user (Hughes & Robertson, 1991). Many youth report that they are more likely to die of gunshot wounds than AIDS and as a result, they do not see any reason to take precautions (Waters et al., 1996). The selected sites of welfare hotels, welfare offices, Teen Progress and the Essex County Youth House Detention Center service populations who have had difficulty with authority, social mores, and obtaining the essentials needed to live a safe and healthy life. In order to illuminate the level of resistance to be anticipated in the population at the Essex County Youth Detention Center, we refer the reader to an incident reported in *The New York Times* (Nieves, 1996). Dr. Joe Clarke (famous as the former principal of East Side High School depicted in the film *Lean on Me*), director of the center, felt compelled to shackle some of the youth to their beds due to their dangerous and disruptive behavior (e.g., attacking guards and other detainees and throwing urine and feces around the facility). Some of the clients were awaiting trial for drug dealing, assault, and murder. A few feared being remanded to criminal court to be tried as adults. In one particular case, the girlfriend of a male detainee who was charged with murder was charged as his accomplice. She was pregnant at the time with his child.

Most programs in Newark have involved primary prevention efforts in public schools. However, there were and continue to be several easily identifiable groups who are at very high risk for contracting AIDS, including adolescents in the criminal justice system, teenage mothers, and welfare families who would not be exposed to traditional programs in the educational system.

The basic premise for CDC-funded programs remains that changes in knowledge, beliefs, and attitudes will eventually lead to changes in behavior, but clearly not without other important components. Given the impact of the prevention literature, participants should also be taught social and negotiation skills. These segments should involve modeling by the facilitators and role playing by the participants. One of the most important components should be the development of individual plans for a productive, self-protective, total lifestyle. Since drug therapeutic communities have already demonstrated an ability to provide effective treatment for drug addicts, it was expected that their counselors would be excellent role models and would have the requisite skills to deal with high-risk populations such as adolescents who are involved in the criminal justice system. Integrity House, a drug therapeutic community in Newark, prepared a program whose primary goal was to change the behavior of high-risk adolescents.

The program was first implemented in 1989 at four basic sites: the Essex County Youth Detention Center, "Teen Progress" (a welfare program for teenage mothers), the Essex County welfare offices, and the Essex County welfare hotels. While the original target group was adolescents, both adolescents and adults were present at the welfare offices and hotels. One of the salient elements that distinguished this program from prior educational efforts that typify other programs across the United States is that the counselors here used the confrontational style developed in the therapeutic community context. The therapeutic community model has been used with the drug-addicted population since the 1950s. The primary goal of the therapeutic community is to foster personal growth by changing the individual's personal lifestyle within a community of concerned people working together to help themselves and each other. Through the use of treatment community-imposed sanctions and penalties as well as earned advancement of status and privileges as part of the recovery and growth process, members progress and begin to see changes in one another (DeLeon 1988).

PREVENTION

The staff for the program were recruited in two different searches one through a newspaper advertisement and the second by word of mouth. During the interview process, applicants were asked about their ability and comfort level with group presentations and their perspectives on (1) people that are utilizing the welfare system, (2) teenage pregnancy, (3) homelessness, and (4) juvenile delinquency. The staff members who had the longest retention record within the prevention program, the strongest rapport with the participants, and who were able to adapt to each of the different locations were the ones who had first-hand experience with one or more of the social issues listed above. The staffing for the program included peer educators who were to be scheduled on a part-time basis and full-time health educators who were to be paired as cofacilitators. The peer educators who were hired had almost identical early personal histories to the youth at the detention center and the young women at Teen Progress and were extremely successful in their delivery and served as role models. The program director and the external evaluator evaluated the performance of staff members on a regular basis. Full-time staff who had empathy for the populations but had little or no first-hand knowledge of the community did not last very long in the program. It is uncertain if the differences in backgrounds prevented the clients from establishing rapport and giving respect and trust to the workers or if the workers were unable to understand the needs of the clients. The answer is probably a combination of both factors.

The most effective staff members seemed to be the facilitators who were themselves seropositive and "recovering" from drug addictions. Even when they chose not to reveal their status, the prevention educators' messages were passionately and credibly delivered and stressed the importance of thinking before choosing actions that may be unsafe. While each team's sessions were guided by a script, the facilitators were able to respond effectively to spontaneous challenges from the participants. Therapeutic community philosophy emphasizes confronting irrational attitudes and beliefs (DeLeon, 1988). Many of the prevention program staff were actually graduates of Integrity House which means that they had experienced the same process themselves and could demonstrate what they themselves had learned. Therapeutic communities also believe in the concept of rational authority, respect for others, and safety and security in one's environment, all of which enhanced the program and enabled participants to develop problem-solving skills.

In designing this program, we remembered that no theory is better than its implementation. Attention to detail is important. For example, since being a role model was a component of the program, even the appropriateness of attire was considered. However, the strict dress code used for work within Integrity would have been completely unsuitable. Business attire would have lent an air of superiority to the staff that would have interfered with its message and created a "we-they" dichotomy. Consequently, employees wore street clothes (jeans and sneakers) which assisted them in putting the clients at ease and allowed the workers "to be themselves" and respond to the clients on an equal level. The language style of each presentation was also important. "Street talk" in reference to sexual intercourse, drugs, relationships, and crime was utilized to assure that the proper information was being communicated to the participants.

Each program component also used ethnically sensitive and age appropriate media presentations, discussion group topics, and role plays to sensitize clients to the seriousness of HIV transmission. The media selections were chosen from ETS Associates and CDC lists available to HIV prevention programs. To assure good communication and a realistic evaluation of the program, questionnaires were designed at a 4th grade reading level, translated to Spanish, and read to clients as needed for comprehension. The questions tapped changes in knowledge, attitudes, perceived risk level, beliefs and reported behaviors There were 16 questions for each session. The research design involved pretesting and posttesting the participants on the content of that session

There were both similarities and differences among the program components at the various sites that need to be described. At the Youth Detention Center, all the detainees were included. The teams repeated the presentations at each unit. The center has three floors and two units per floor. Each unit generally contains 20-30 youth. At the Essex County Youth Detention Center, four sessions (two hours each) were conducted over a period of four weeks. The detainees were mandated to attend. The only times that they were allowed to miss sessions were either for health reasons or court-related matters.

The "Teen Progress" program addressed the problems of approximately fifty pregnant young women who were outpatients. They were divided into two groups. For the Teen Progress program, Essex county policy stated that these young mothers must be required to participate or their welfare checks would be reduced. The clients at Teen Progress were exposed to two sessions per week for three weeks. Thus, there was a strong element of coercion at both of the adolescent facilities.

The number of people in the Welfare hotels and offices at any single session was highly variable, ranging from as few as two to approximately 100. The presentations at the welfare offices were conducted in the waiting room. A single session lasted for two hours and people were free to leave at any time. The people at the welfare hotels were notified over the public address systems that there would be a movie about HIV prevention and that condoms would be distributed. Again participation was strictly on a volunteer basis. This latter presentation also took two hours. At the welfare hotels, cookies and nonalcoholic punch were served as an inducement to attend. Reading materials were distributed at each site.

All presentations challenged the irrational thinking and maladaptive behavioral practices of the participants. The message in the first session at the youth detention center and "Teen Progress," was essentially that "AIDS is a disease that kills and that it is spread by sharing needles and having unprotected sex. The client is likely to catch it if he or she does not use protection." The pretest questionnaires tapped the reasons why an adolescent might *not* take precautions against AIDS as well as real knowledge about sexual practices. The posttest focused on information in the presentation that addressed the pretest issues. It also assessed change in perceived level of risk. It was assumed that without an awareness of the risk factors, no one would be motivated to make the necessary changes in behavior. The largest numbers of participants were exposed to that single session since it was also presented at the welfare offices and hotels.

The second, third, and fourth sessions were given only to adolescents at the youth house and at Teen Progress. The second session emphasized safer sex practices as well as the development of the social skills necessary to negotiate safer sex with a partner. The third session centered on how people use drugs and alcohol to avoid dealing with problems and feelings and how substance abuse puts the individual at risk for contracting AIDS. The questionnaire included drug abuse information and measured attitudes concerning alcohol and drug use. In the fourth session, the participants were required to develop a realistic plan of action to avoid infection and to establish a productive lifestyle. The following section deals with the research aspect of the program.

METHOD

Participants

The total number of clients served was at all sites 3,460. Of those, 514 adolescents, who were almost all male (n = 495), were detained in the Youth House, 162 were adolescent women in the Teen Progress program; and 2,536 were individuals at the welfare sites (males, n = 216; females, n = 2,320).

Not all the adolescents either in the youth detention center or in Teen Progress were exposed to the complete series of presentations. Some of the adolescents in the youth detention center may only have been exposed to the first and second sessions of the program and then

may have left because their cases were adjudicated. Completely differ
ent detainees may have finished the third and fourth sessions (o:
variations of the above patterns). At the welfare sites, people were free
to come in late (no pretest), and may have been called away early (nc
posttest). There may also be "repeaters" at the welfare sites. Partici
pants were only identified by birth date and city. The questionnaire:
themselves are anonymous.

Procedure

At each session, an attempt was made to collect both pretest anc
posttest data, although not necessarily from the same clients, as wc
previously noted. It was possible to separate the sets. The question·
naires tapped three areas of functioning: (1) Knowledge about AIDS
sexual behavior, and drugs and alcohol; (2) attitudes towards sexua
behavior, and drug and alcohol use; and (3) self-reports of behavior
self-esteem, and personal experiences including perceived behavior o
friends and family. Perceived level of risk was also assessed.

RESULTS AND DISCUSSION

The analyses utilized the pretest/posttest comparisons of the dat;
from subjects who filled out both questionnaires for the first session a:
well as some "pretest only" or "posttest only" information. The
reason that we included these questionnaires is that we thought we
might have a natural Solomon four group design. The independen:
variables were sex of participant, age category (under 22, over 22)
and racial/ethnic group (Black, White, and Hispanic). The "other'
category was dropped from the analysis since it was too heteroge·
neous to be useful (i.e., it included Asian Americans, Native Ameri·
cans, and individuals who identified themselves as both Black anc
Hispanic, etc.).

In Session 1, utilizing the entire sample (N = 2,453), the reader wil
see that we can easily conclude that both adolescents and adults have
already been exposed to most of the information presently available
concerning HIV prevention and AIDS. Consequently, the data are pri·
marily from the pretest unless otherwise specified. For example, on the
statement, "A person can get AIDS from sharing needles used to injeci
drugs," 97.9 percent of the adolescents and 97.3 percent of the adult:

were correct in knowing that sharing needles is dangerous. It is actually quite surprising to see that 2.5 percent of the total sample did not grasp that fact even after the intervention. The so-called adults were included because they were predominantly young women with young children.

Again on the pretest, both adolescents and adults agreed (97.1 percent and 98.4 percent respectfully) that " . . . teenagers can get AIDS." The questions were based on a list of myths including the idea that teenagers cannot get AIDS. While the reader may find such a myth incredible, please believe that at one time that concept had been expressed by many of the youth with whom we worked in Newark. Fortunately, times have changed. Similar percentages of the participant groups (96.9 percent and 97.8 percent) acknowledged that "a pregnant woman who has AIDS (the HIV virus) can pass it to her unborn child."

When asked if "A person can be HIV infected and not show signs of the disease," 83 percent of the adolescents and 87.5 percent of the adults knew that it is possible to appear asymptomatic and still be HIV positive. Approximately 80 percent of the adolescents and 87 percent of the adults knew that "there is a connection between drug and alcohol use and sex" (also prior to the presentation). Those answers improved 10.7 percent and 7.4 percent respectively after the sessions, but still did not include the entire group. While we did not expect 100 percent concurrence, this point was continually emphasized and remained a disappointment.

Before the session, only 18.5 percent of the adolescents and 20.7 percent of the adults understood that a person could still "get AIDS from having sex using a condom (rubber)." The presentation is very clear that the only guarantee for not becoming infected is abstinence and that condoms have a failure rate. Almost 47 percent of the teenagers and 52 percent of the adults continued to maintain that condoms give total protection from HIV. It is important that people understand that condoms are not completely safe and that, in fact, it matters which condoms are used and how they are used. We must work on this issue.

Given the importance of risk as a motivating factor, participants were asked to assess their personal chances of getting AIDS. Unfortunately, the results indicate that even after the presentation and despite information readily available in the media and from other reliable sources to the contrary, this sample does not essentially see itself as being at high risk for HIV infection. It is clear from an examination of the table depicting reported self perceptions of risk for acquiring HIV that in all conditions (Pretest Only, Posttest Only, and Pretest/Posttes complete sets), the participants essentially evaluated themselves a being either at no risk or low risk (see Table 1). Consequently, thei level of risk is increased. It was the contention of the program that ar awareness of one's personal danger would enhance the desire to devel op a more self-protective lifestyle. On the other hand, we did not wan the participants to feel hopeless. Some anxiety is motivating; too mucl is debilitating. The chi-square analyses indicated significant difference: in their perception of risk between the Pretest Only and Posttest Onl) groups (Chi Square = 23.57, df = 4, p = .05), with the Posttest Onl) participants reporting that they perceived themselves to be at higher risl than the Pretest Only participants. This finding, which emerged early ir the project, led us to question whether or not taking the pretest migh actually have contaminated the intervention process. We hypothesizec that once the members of the audience had stated that they were a "no" or "low risk," it was quite possible that they denied or resistec the message of the intervention. A comparison of the posttests for twc groups (Posttest Only and Pretest/Posttest), however, indicated no sig nificant differences. We noted that the participants who completed botl

TABLE 1. Responses to the question, "What are your chances of getting AIDS?" (N = 2453).

Participants	Perceived chances of getting AIDS					
	High	Medium	Low	None	No Answer	Total
Pretest only (and then left)	n = 79 (14.8%)	49 (9.2%)	110 (20.7%)	231 (43.5%)	62 (11. 6%)	531
Posttest only (came late)	38 (16%)	29 (12.2%)	75 (31.6%)	66 (27.8%)	29 (12.2%)	237
Complete Sets (both pretest and posttest)						
Pretest	258 (15.3%)	211 (12.5%)	440 (26%)	607 (36%)	169 (10%)	1685
Posttest	230 (13.6%)	232 (13.7%)	480 (28%)	566 (33.5%)	177 (10.5%)	Same

questionnaires along with the intervention seemed to see themselves as being at higher risk initially than those in the Pretest Only condition; that may help to explain the results. Since they were interspersed among all the workshops, there is no reason to suppose that they were qualitatively different from the other participants prior to the intervention. Although, due to the fact that the Pretest Only participants did not complete the intervention or the posttest procedure, one might be led to believe that they were even more resistant than the rest of the sample. They may simply have left the presentation.

Much to our surprise, there were no significant differences on any of the questions by age or by sex of participant. The numbers of White and Hispanic participants were insufficient to conduct meaningful racial comparisons. However, there was a very slight tendency for Hispanic adult males to see themselves as being at lower risk than all other groups and for Hispanic women to perceive themselves at higher risk than all other groups.

In terms of evaluating the overall efficacy of this and other HIV prevention programs, we must place these efforts in context and examine several factors. We do know that education once helped the high-risk gay population (especially in San Francisco) to reduce the number of new cases. We do know that the participants in this program were either already aware of important facts about AIDS before the presentations or learned the necessary information during the sessions, but that they continued to deny their own high level of risk. There may, of course, be several reasons that account for the perceived low risk. Besides engaging in denial, they may actually be taking some precautions (although informal interviews indicated that they do not use condoms), or they may think that they already have AIDS. Another and perhaps more critical explanation for low perceived risk concerns attitudes toward the possibility of dying from AIDS as compared to dying from the other threats in Newark. Adolescents in inner cities see themselves as being in danger of being killed before they are 21 from gunshot wounds or other types of violence. They don't see AIDS as the most immediate threat. They may say to themselves "If I'm going to die, I might as well live the way I want to right now." Thus, the factors that must be changed before both adolescents and adults can benefit from HIV prevention programs are monumental.

CONCLUSION

There is no doubt that it is difficult to develop effective prevention programs for hard-to-reach-populations and that positive results are troublesome to demonstrate, but the fight continues. For professional in this field, there is sufficient HIV prevention work to do so tha adding to the burden with other issues seems unfair. However, it is ou contention (and that of many others such as Wilson, 1996; and Samp son et al., 1997) that if we do not attempt to address other ills ii society, our youth will never believe that they have a stake in the future. It is apparent, for example, that the adolescents in the Youtl Detention Center, many of whom will be remanded to adult court would have great difficulty in believing any message about the pur pose of using condoms. Many of us will have to become advocates fo changes in the school system, for vocational training, for economi opportunities, better housing, and other social changes or the minima interventions we are attempting are doomed from the beginning. I was not our purpose to focus only on the needs of minorities in the inner cities. Many adolescents from all racial, ethnic, and economi groups share the same propensities for risk taking. One need only lool at the increases in smoking in adolescents across the country to se that high-risk behavior cuts across social categories.

With respect to this study and the prevention program upon which i is based, we can speak mainly to the need for careful selection o credible leaders who can serve as both role models and experts. Ther are ample appropriate audio-visual support materials from which to choose as well. Without disregarding the knowledge components, the development of a sense of self-efficacy and the acquisition of prob lem-solving and negotiating skills is critical. Throughout the program the motivation for change must be reinforced. What concerns us the most about any minimal intervention is the need for follow-up anc relapse prevention (return to one's former dysfunctional lifestyle) Since there probably won't be a sufficient number of supportive adult who can mentor our youth in need, the question remains how can we strengthen the youth of America (or around the world for that matter in the face of a hostile environment. The public must be encouraged to examine policy and to take responsibility for future generations re gardless of whose children they are.

REFERENCES

Amaro, H. (1995). Love sex and power: Considering women's realities in HIV prevention. *American Psychologist, 50*(6), 437-447.

Amaro, H., Zuckerman, B., Cabal, J. (1989). Drug use among adolescent mothers: Profiles of risk. *Pediatrics, 84*, 144-151.

Bandura, A. (1988). Perceived self-efficacy in the exercise of control over AIDS infection. In V.M, Albee, G.W. & S. F. Schneider (Eds.), *Primary prevention of AIDS: Psychological* approaches (pp. 128-141). Newbury Park, CA: SAGE Publications, Inc.

Bennett, W. S., Dilulio, J. J., & Walters, J. P., (1997). *Body count.* New York: Simon and Schuster.

Boatler, J. F., Knight, K., & Simpson, D. D. (1994). Assessment of an AIDS intervention program during substance abuse treatment. *Journal of Substance Abuse Treatment, 11*(4), 367-372.

Boyer, C. B., & Ellen, J. M. (1994). HIV risk in adolescents: The role of sexual activity and substance abuse behaviors. In Battjes, R. J., Sloboda, Z., & Grace, W. C. (Eds.), *The context of HIV risk among drug users and their sexual partners* (pp. 135-154). Rockville, MD: US Department of Health and Human Services. National Institute on Drug Abuse Research Monograph #143.

Boyer, C. B., Shafer, M., & Tschann, J. M. (1997). Evaluation of a knowledge and cognitive behavioral skills-building intervention to prevent STDs and HIV infection in high school students. *Adolescence, 32*(125), 25-42.

Center for Disease Control. (1997, December 31). *HIV/AIDS surveillance report.* Atlanta, Georgia [On-line], Available: www.cdc.gov.

Center for Substance Abuse Prevention. (1992). *Quick list: Ten steps to a drug-free future* (DHHS Publication No. (ADM) 92). Rockville, MD: US Department of Health and Human Services.

Chubb, N. H., Fertan, C. I., & Ross, J. L. (1997). Adolescent self-esteem and locus of control: A longitudinal study of gender and age differences. *Adolescence, 32*(125), 113-129.

DeLeon, G. (1988). The therapeutic community perspective and approach for adolescent substance abusers. In Feinstein, S. (Ed.), *Adolescent psychiatry* (pp. 535-557). Chicago: University of Chicago.

Division of STD Prevention (September, 1996). *Sexually transmitted disease surveillance, 1995.* U.S. Department of Health and Human Services, Public Health Service. Atlanta: Centers for Disease Control and Prevention. [On-line], Available: Http://wonder.cdc.gov/rchtml/convert/std/cstd3815/pcw.html

Farber, J. Waters, J., Levine, L., & Hennen, J. (1995). *Childhood abuse in relationship to substance abuse in adolescence.* Paper presented at the Eastern Psychological Association meeting, Boston, MA.

Green, J. (1996, September 15). Just say no? *The New York Times Magazine*, pp. 39-45, 54-55, 84-85.

Greene, K., Hale, J. L., & Rubin, D. L. (1997). A test of the theory of reasoned action in the context of condom use and AIDS. *Communications Reports, 10*(1), 21-33.

Hughes, K., & Robertson, J. G. (1991). *Programs against drug abuse and the spread of AIDS: Contributions of the drug therapeutic community approach.* Paper presented at the meeting of the Eastern Psychological Association, New York, Nev York.

Katz, R. C., Mills, K., Singh, N. N., & Best, A. M. (1995). Knowledge and attitude: about AIDS: A comparison of public high school students, incarcerated delin quents, and emotionally disturbed adolescents. *Journal of Youth and Adolescence* *24*(1), 117-131.

Lombardi, E., Cargill, V., Stephens, R., & Gigliotti, R. (1997). *The effect of socia networks upon the HIV risk behavior of adolescent African-American females* [On-line]

Luker, K. (1996). *Dubious conceptions? The politics of teenage pregnancy.* Cam bridge, MA: Harvard University Press.

Martin, D. (1997, November 3). N.Y. Man accused of spreading HIV appears ir court. *Infoseek News Channel* [On-line], xx. Available: www.infoseek.com.

Mills, C., Turner, C., & Moses, L. (Eds.). (1990). *AIDS: The second decade.* Wash ington, DC: National Academy Press.

Morton, M., Nelson, L., Walsh C., Zimmerman, S. & Coe, R. M. (1996). Evaluatior of an HIV/AIDS education program for adolescents. *Journal of Communit; Health, 21*(1), 23-35.

New Jersey State Department of Health (1997, June 30). New Jersey HIV/AIDS Cases. Trenton, NJ.

Nieves, E. (1996, September 20). Disciplinarian is not sorry for shackling. *The Nev York Times*, p. L. 39.

Post, S. G., & Botkin, J. R. (1995). Adolescents and AIDS prevention: The Pediatri cian's Role. *Clinical Pediatrics, 34*(1), 41-46.

Prochaska, J. O., DiClemente, C. C. & Norcross, J.C. (1992). In search of how peopl change: Applications to addictive behaviors. *American Psychologist, 47*(9) 1102-1114.

Reuters (10/27/97). *NY Officials say at least 11 HIV cases traced to man.* Infoseel News Channel [On-line], xx. Available: www.infoseek.com/news1486

Roberts, A. R., & Waters, J. A. (1998). The coming storm. In A. R. Roberts (Ed.) *Juvenile justice.* (pp. 40-70). New York, Nelson Hall.

Robertson, J. G., & Waters, J. A. (1994). Inner city adolescents and drug abuse. In A R. Roberts (Ed.), *Critical issues in crime and justice* (pp. 171-188). London: Sag Publications.

Romer, D., & Kim, S. (1995). Health interventions for African Americans and Latinc youth: The potential role of mass media. *Health Education Quarterly, 22* 172-189.

Sampson, R. J., Raudenbush, S. W., & Earls, F. (1997). Neighborhoods and violen crime: A multilevel study of collective efficacy. *Science, 277*, 918-924.

Sexton, J. (1997, October 10). From bad child to one-man epidemic, suspect i: recalled as out of control. *New York Times* [On-line], Available: www.nytimes com.

Sullivan, R. T. (1996). The challenge of HIV prevention among high-risk adoles cents. [On-line]. *Health and Social Work*, 21(1), 58-65. Article from: Ebscohost.

U.S. Department of Health and Human Services (1991). *Healthy people 2000.* Atlan ta: U.S. Department of Health and Human Services.

Waters, J. Roberts, A. R., & Morgen K. (1997). High-risk pregnancies: Teenagers, poverty, and drug abuse. *Journal of Drug Issues, 27*(3), 541-562.

Waters, J. A., Morgen, K., Kuttner, P. V., Schmitt, B., & Schwartz, A. (1996). The "guiding adolescents to prevention" program: Reducing HIV transmission and drug use in youth in a detention center. *Crisis Intervention, 3,* 86-96.

Wilson, W. J. (1996, Aug. 18). Work. *The New York Times Magazine,* 26-30, 40, 48, 52-54.

Wulfertead, B. A. (1994). A contextual approach to research on AIDS prevention. *The Behavior Analyst, 17*(2), 353-363.

Minors' Rights and HIV:
Prevention, Testing and Treatment

Thera M. Meehan
Kevin Cranston

SUMMARY. This article will examine the concept of minors' legal rights and their relationship to HIV prevention, HIV counseling and testing, and the treatment of HIV infection. The legal concept of minors' rights being equal to adults' legal rights has emerged in the last three decades. Parallel to this emergence is the changing nature of child/adolescent morbidity and mortality. Significant increases in rates of suicide, drug use, sexually transmitted diseases (STDs), violent crimes, and births to single adolescent mothers have occurred over the same time period. More recently, there has been a rapid increase in the number of reported AIDS cases in the adolescent age group (13-19 years), which includes minors. It could be argued that this reflects a society in which minors practice behaviors more characteristic of adults. If so, a right to access services related to these behaviors should be granted to minors, specifically as they relate to HIV infection. *[Article copies available for a fee from The Haworth Document Delivery Service: 1-800-342-9678. E-mail address: getinfo@haworthpressinc.com]*

KEYWORDS. Minors, HIV, AIDS, legal issues, prevention, testing, treatment

Thera M. Meehan, MSW, MPH, is Senior Health Policy Analyst, Massachusetts Department of Public Health, HIV/AIDS Bureau, 250 Washington Street, Boston, MA 02108 (e-mail: thera.meehan@state.ma.us).

Kevin Cranston, MDiv, is Director, Prevention and Education Services, Massachusetts Department of Public Health, HIV/AIDS Bureau, 250 Washington Street, Boston, MA 02108 (e-mail: kevin.cranston@state.ma.us).

[Haworth co-indexing entry note]: "Minors' Rights and HIV: Prevention, Testing and Treatment." Meehan, Thera M. and Kevin Cranston. Co-published simultaneously in *Journal of HIV/AIDS Prevention & Education for Adolescents & Children* (The Haworth Press, Inc.) Vol. 3, No. 1/2, 1999, pp. 79-98; and: *HIV Affected and Vulnerable Youth: Prevention Issues and Approaches* (ed: Susan Taylor-Brown and Alejandro Garcia) The Haworth Press, Inc., 1999, pp. 79-98. Single or multiple copies of this article are available for a fee from The Haworth Document Delivery Service [1-800-342-9678, 9:00 a.m. - 5:00 p.m. (EST). E-mail address: getinfo@haworthpressinc.com].

© 1999 by The Haworth Press, Inc. All rights reserved.

Since the inception of diagnosed AIDS case reporting by the Centers for Disease Control and Prevention (CDC), 3,130 cases of AIDS
have been reported in the adolescent age category (13-19 years old)
(CDC, 1997). AIDS in adolescents was first diagnosed, retrospective-
ly, in 1981 (Vermund et al., 1989). Since that time, the number of
reported cases in adolescents has seen yearly increases. In 1994, 1,965
cumulative AIDS cases were reported in adolescents (CDC, 1994).
This increased to 2,354 cases in 1995 (CDC, 1995), and to 2,754 in
1996 (CDC, 1996).

The majority of adolescent AIDS cases in the U.S. are in males
(62%). The risk category "hemophilia/coagulation disorder" continues to account for a large portion of cases (23%), but it is closely
followed by "heterosexual contact" (22%) and "men who have sex
with men" (21%) (CDC, 1997). A small, yet alarming, percentage of
adolescents (10%) fall in the "injecting drug use" risk category. A
review of the risk associated with reported AIDS cases in the 20-24
year age category reflects risk behaviors practiced during adolescence
as an adolescent may be infected with HIV at a young age but not
reported as an AIDS case for several years. The risk reported in this
age category is very different from that of the adolescent age category
Of the 22,953 cases in the 20-24 year age group, almost half fall in the
"men who have sex with men" (46%) risk category. This is followed
by "injecting drug use" (17%), "heterosexual contact" (17%), and
"men who have sex with men and inject drugs" (8%) (CDC, 1997).

Almost 50% of reported adolescent AIDS cases are identified as
Black, 32% as White, and 19% as Hispanic. African Americans and
Hispanics represent close to 25% of the total U.S. population, yet in
adolescents, these groups represent 56% of AIDS cases reported in
males, and 82% of AIDS cases reported in females (CDC, 1998). A
growing percentage of adolescent AIDS cases were infected with HIV
perinatally. Advances in identification and treatment of infection have
led to prolonged survival (Grubman et al., 1995).

The reporting of HIV infection, distinct from AIDS case reporting,
further illustrates that HIV infection has penetrated the adolescent
population. Through 1997, 3,574 cases of HIV infection in adolescents have been reported to the CDC (CDC, 1997). Since HIV reporting is mandated in only 29 states, this figure represents only a portion
of HIV infection in the adolescent age category in the U.S. Certain
projection models indicate that the age of onset of HIV infection is

occurring at much younger ages (Rosenberg, Biggar & Goedert, 1994).

Adolescents are clearly at risk for HIV infection. Within the adolescent population a legal distinction is drawn between minors and those 18 years of age and older. In certain contexts, such as HIV infection, referring to adolescents without applying the legal distinction of minors complicates the discussion as legal rights within the adolescent category vary by age. Many government agencies define adolescents as ages 13-21 years (D'Angelo, 1992). From a legal perspective, which is acknowledged when considering HIV prevention education, testing and treatment, 18-21 years olds have rights that differ from 13-17 year olds. These rights may vary further by state.

The legal concept of children's rights being equal to adults' legal rights has emerged only in the last three decades (Plotkin, 1981). Parallel to this emergence is the changing nature of adolescent morbidity and mortality. Significant increases in rates of suicide, drug use, sexually transmitted diseases (STDs), violent crimes and births to single adolescent mothers have occurred over the same time period (AMA, 1993). This trend, we argue, reflects a society in which adolescents practice behaviors more characteristic of adults (Holder, 1987). If so, a right to access services related to these behaviors should be granted to adolescents, including minors.

MINORS' RIGHTS AND THE LAW

The Supreme Court has noted, "Constitutional rights do not mature and come into being only when one attains the state-defined age of majority. Minors, as well as adults, are protected by the Constitution and possess constitutional rights" (Sigman & O'Connor, 1991, p. 522). Historically, rights bestowed during adolescence are done so by degrees corresponding with age. They have not necessarily reflected adolescent life circumstances or events.

When we refer to minors' rights, we are generally referring to minors' right to consent to a variety of treatment-related services, as well as rights to be exposed to or disclose certain types of information. In the context of HIV infection and AIDS, we are referring to minors' right to consent to certain health-related services: prevention education services, counseling and testing, and treatment. Under U.S. law, minors have been traditionally deemed incompetent to consent, or

give informed consent, for health care. This common law rule sug
gests that consent of a minor's parent or guardian is necessary t
obtain health care services (Wing, 1992; Holder, 1977). It is presume
that the law regards minors as incompetent to consent to health car
services because they are lacking the capacity to make logical deci
sions. The rationale for the requirement of parental consent, then, i
one of protection of the minor from making rash decisions (Gittle
Quigley-Rich & Saks, 1990).

The notion of parental notification differs from parental consent i
its association with the principle of confidentiality. In the realm c
health care services, confidentiality has been recognized in the clini
cian-patient relationship (Gittler, Quigley-Rich & Saks, 1990). Th
principle of confidentiality requires that health care providers nc
reveal information about a patient without the consent of the patier
(Annas, 1993). Courts and legislatures through certain privileges asso
ciated with the clinician-patient relationship have historically prc
tected confidentiality.

Exceptions to the parental consent rule have emerged in U.S. law
The American Medical Association (AMA) realized as early as 196
that to prevent the spread of STDs, minors needed access to car
without parental consent (Holder, 1988). Most state statutes also au
thorize minors to consent to pregnancy care, alcohol and drug us
treatment (AMA, 1993), as well as medical care in an emergenc
situation (although the definition of emergency differs from state t
state) (Sigman & O'Connor, 1991). Rights granted to minors concern
ing health care originate from a recognition of the balance of minors
liberty and privacy interests with the interests of the state (Henggele
Melton & Rodgrigue, 1992). The Supreme Court ruled in 1977 tha
minors have a right of privacy which encompasses contraceptio
(Holder, 1987).

Occasionally, when consent from a parent or guardian was no
required, courts and legislatures replaced the rule with that of parenta
notification. This was done with a similar rationale to that of parenta
consent (Gittler, Quigley-Rich & Saks, 1990). From the viewpoint of
minor, parental notification may not be distinguishable from parenta
consent (English, 1990).

The common law principles of "emancipated minors" and "matur
minors" represent exceptions to the parental consent rule and gran
minors the right to act on their own behalf (Holder, 1988). "Emanci

pated minors" refers to those minors who possess legal rights of adulthood, specifically married minors, minors in the armed forces, unmarried minor mothers, minors living apart from their parents, or minors managing their own financial affairs (English, 1990). "Mature minors" refers to those minors who have received a legal judgment as to whether the minor understands the proposed health care service, including its risk and benefits (AMA, 1993).

One may argue that minors have a right to access or consent to health-related services, or certain types of health-related services, as if they were adults. Access to health care is obviously particularly important during adolescence as this is a time of exploration of new behaviors, and the availability of health-related services may help educate and modify risk behaviors. However, adolescents, including minors, continue to face barriers to gaining access to health services.

Findings from a study of adolescent health by the Office of Technology Assessment (OTA) indicated that adolescents face barriers, especially to early intervention services, due to geographic factors, lack of health insurance, lack of adolescent-specific providers, and lack of knowledge (Dougherty, 1993). Confidentiality has also been identified as a barrier to services and care for adolescents. Uncertainty about whether services will be confidential leads some adolescents to avoid care altogether, or suppress sensitive information once they have sought care (AMA, 1993).

It is clear that courts and legislatures have attempted to respond to the changing nature of health issues in adolescents. Adolescents, and minors, have been granted more freedom to exercise their rights to access and consent to health care services. Certain rights bestowed to minors have been tested, and continue to be tested, as minors are forced to address the HIV epidemic. The following sections address minors' rights as they relate to this epidemic, specifically examining prevention education, HIV antibody counseling and testing, and treatment.

HIV PREVENTION

HIV prevention services represent an arena where minors' rights may be the least clear as prevention services are presented in a variety of ways, and may therefore be accessed in a variety of ways. Prevention services may be accessed at school, through peers, at community-based clinics or agencies, in physicians' offices, or through the media.

Perhaps the most prominent form of prevention services for minors is school-based health education. In most states, young people are required to be in school until age 16, often before the initiation of risk-taking behaviors. Health education has long been a part of the curriculum for many school systems across the country. As the recognition of HIV infection in the adolescent population became more prominent, many school systems incorporated safe sex and HIV prevention messages into existing health education curriculum (Kirby 1992).

The decision to implement school-based HIV prevention programs originates generally in the local board of education, or with the superintendent of schools. National polls taken in the 1980s revealed that parents and adolescents alike supported sexuality education and HIV prevention programs (Norman & Harris, 1981; Leo, Delany & Whitaker, 1986). Twenty-two states and the District of Columbia require some form of sexuality education and STD/HIV prevention education Fifteen states require only STD/HIV prevention education, and 13 states do not require either one (NARAL, 1995). The greatest barrier to the implementation of sexuality education and HIV prevention programs in schools originates from groups of parents, conservative community groups, or members of the school administration (Kirby 1992). Inadequate funding and policy decisions also affect the implementation of these programs.

The majority of state boards of education or local school districts support or mandate sexuality education and HIV prevention education, yet not all programs are comprehensive, sources of contraception are not always addressed, and the education is not always delivered at appropriate grade levels. Many school systems begin sexuality education and HIV prevention education in high school, a time after which many students have initiated sexual intercourse (Marsiglio & Mott 1986).

The literature tells us exposure to HIV prevention education does not necessarily translate into practice. Adolescents are knowledgeable about HIV infection and AIDS, but do not always alter risky behaviors (Walter et al., 1992; Keller et al., 1991; Holtzman et al., 1992). Some degree of risk-taking is developmentally appropriate for adolescents Some adolescents also experience a lack of access to prevention devices, such as condoms.

The use of condoms as a device to prevent HIV infection has been supported by the CDC since the onset of the AIDS epidemic (CDC, 1993a). Access to condoms is not consistent across age groups, and may be more difficult for minors, due to cost or the social stigma associated with their purchase, and the inherent difficulty of negotiating their use.

The Supreme Court has recognized minors' right to access contraception including condoms (*Carey v. Population Services International, 1977*). Many school systems have recognized this right through the advent of school-based condom availability programs. To date, more than 400 schools in the United States have implemented condom availability programs (Guttmacher et al., 1997). These programs have not emerged or existed without controversy. School-based condom availability programs test the rights of parents to control the upbringing of their children. Although many parents support these programs (Guttmacher et al., 1995), many parents and community groups see condom availability programs as an infringement on their parental rights.

In 1993, a Massachusetts school district was challenged legally for instituting a condom availability program. A community group challenged the local school committee on several different grounds. The group charged that the condom availability program infringed on family privacy and free exercise rights; functioned as an accomplice to statutory rape on or by the students; promoted and failed to report sexual abuse of minors using condoms; and was in violation of the moral education statute (*Curtis v. The Falmouth School Committee*).

The central theme of the case involved the competing interest of parents and the school committee in the education of children. This theme parallels the concept discussed earlier, that minors are incompetent and need the protection of parents (or guardians) or others (school committees) to make decisions.

The Massachusetts Superior Court upheld the school committee's condom availability policy as constitutional. The Court made a clear distinction between "condom availability" and "condom distribution," by expressing the view that "condom availability" is not coercive and allows parents or guardians to exercise control over their minor children. Minors' rights to access condoms in school in this case were ultimately protected. Similar cases in the cities of New York (*Alfonso v. Fernandez and the Board of Education for the City of New York, 1992*) and Philadelphia (*Harold Stephens and Philip Battaglia v. School*

District of the Philadelphia Board of Education. et al., 1992) also found that parents' rights had not been violated and upheld the right of minors to access condoms in schools.

Although adolescents report that most of their HIV/AIDS preven tion education is received in school, the media is also a source o information (Guttmacher et al., 1995). Minors' rights to be exposed t(HIV prevention messages through the media vary by parent, guardian community and the availability of HIV prevention messages in loca media.

Media-based prevention efforts have not been studied as vigorousl as school-based prevention programs. An examination of White an(Latino adolescents found both to have substantial exposure to AID.' education information through the media, especially print media an(radio. Of note, White adolescents had greater exposure to AIDS infor mation and condom use, while Hispanic adolescents had greater expo sure to the risk of injection drug use (Hofstetter et al., 1995). Thes(differing rates of exposure to prevention messages may account fo differing rates of reported risk behaviors and reported AIDS cases i1 these two ethnic groups.

The impact of one media event that was studied in adults and adoles cents was the announcement by Earvin "Magic" Johnson that he wa infected with HIV. Magic Johnson noted that he wanted to alert youn; +people in particular to the dangers of unsafe sex (CDC, 1993b). Studie varied in their reports of the impact of Magic Johnson's announcement One study of inner city youth showed Magic's announcement had littl(effect on the increase of condom use (Stiffman, Cunningham & Dore 1993). Another study found that 16-24-year-olds did not reduce thei number of sex partners after his announcement (CDC, 1993b). Howevei one study of 12-19-year-old clinic attendees found modest increases i1 awareness of AIDS and intended condom use. Those who were mos influenced by this media event, however, were those who reported th(least risk behaviors (Brown et al., 1996).

HIV prevention messages must be tailored to specific groups as risl behaviors vary and may be influenced by gender and cultural factor: The impact of Magic Johnson's disclosure, for instance, may have ha(greater impact on male heterosexual adolescents. Female adolescent may respond more to HIV prevention messages that are coupled witl pregnancy prevention messages. Among adolescents reported with HI\ infection (not AIDS), the majority of infection reported in male.

was reported in the "men who have sex with men" category. Among female adolescents with HIV, the majority of infection reported is in the "heterosexual contact" category (CDC, 1998). Gender differences may be further complicated by cultural differences. Research has shown that culture may play an important role in the initiation of sex and risky sexual behaviors among Asian/Pacific Islander adolescents (Hou & Basen-Engquist, 1997). In certain cultures, homosexual sex is not tolerated, in particular in young people. This may put pressure on young gay, lesbian, bisexual or transgendered youth to disregard prevention messages and practice unsafe sex in order to hide their sexuality. Prevention messages that do not address cultural and gender stereotypes interfere with successful HIV prevention campaigns.

This broad discussion of access to HIV prevention education messages does not take into account groups within the adolescent population that may be marginalized by society as well as affected by their minor status. These include incarcerated minors, homeless/runaway minors, and gay, lesbian, bisexual and transgendered minors.

Incarcerated minors may face an elevated risk for HIV infection as studies have revealed high rates of STDs in this population (Canterbury et al., 1995). Little research has addressed prevention in this group. Many runaway or street youth come from detention facilities or correctional centers. The complex lifestyle associated with this group of minors makes them difficult to reach. In most states, minors living away from home have the legal rights of adults (English, 1991). Gay, lesbian, bisexual or transgendered youth may be difficult to reach with HIV prevention messages as "coming out" at a young age presents enormous difficulties for some youth. Homophobia and fear of rejection preclude some youth from identifying their sexuality. Certain states, such as Massachusetts, have programs that specifically target the prevention needs of gay/lesbian/bisexual and transgendered youth.

HIV COUNSELING AND TESTING

Testing for HIV antibodies as a component of disease control focuses on individual behavior change as well as slowing the spread of disease in the general population. HIV counseling and testing services may be accessed through primary care physicians, community health centers, STD clinics, pregnancy or prenatal service sites, specific HIV counseling and testing sites, in some school-based clinics, and through

mobile services (such as outreach vans). HIV testing involves exten
sive pre-test and post-test counseling. Recommendations for protocol
for HIV counseling and testing of adolescents have been described in
the literature, with emphasis placed on maintaining the right to confi
dentiality (English, 1989; English, 1991; Futterman et al., 1993). Sero
logic testing of adolescents has been distinguished from that of adults
A blinded unlinked HIV seroprevalence study of adolescents (age
13-19 years) concluded that adolescents infected with HIV may be
overlooked if standard criteria to identify risk are applied to the ado
lescent population (D'Angelo et al., 1991).

Minors' right to consent to HIV counseling and testing is much
more clearly defined than the right to access prevention services. HIV
counseling and testing services provide an opportunity for prevention
messages as well as linkages to services and treatment. With the ad
vent of new life-sustaining HIV treatments, accessing counseling and
testing services is more important than ever.

North (1990) argues that minors may consent to HIV testing in all
states, whether or not explicit statutes exist. This is based on an analy
sis of tort and constitutional law. States vary in their definition of HIV
which governs whether minors may have the right to consent to coun
seling and testing. Minors may also have the right to consent to HIV
testing based on their status as a "mature" or "emancipated" minor
In states where HIV is defined as an STD, minors may consent to HIV
testing and treatment, as statutes exist in all states allowing minors to
consent to STD testing and treatment. Some states define HIV as a
communicable, contagious or infectious disease, or as a mandatory
reportable disease. Minors have the right to consent to HIV testing in
those states based on the definition of HIV (English, 1992; Futterman
Hein & Kunins, 1993; IHPP, 1994). Table 1 presents an overview o
states and their definitions of HIV.

Minors have the right to consent to HIV testing depending upon the
state in which the minor resides. What is less well understood, is
whether or not minors are aware of this right. A study of youth in San
Francisco, Los Angeles, and New York City found that about one-half
of the sample could identify an HIV counseling and testing site (Ro
theram-Borus et al., 1997). The study also found that youth who were
older, identified as homosexual, resided in the West Coast cities, o
had a history of injection drug use were more likely to be tested
Knowledge of HIV testing was not a predictor of seeking testing.

TABLE 1. Minors' Legal Right to Consent to HIV Testing by Statute and Definition of HIV

SPECIFIC STATUTES WHICH ALLOW MINORS TO CONSENT TO HIV TESTING	AZ, CA, CO, CT, DE, IA, MI, MT, NM, NY, OH, WI
SPECIFIC STATUTES WHICH ALLOW MINORS TO CONSENT TO HIV TESTING AND TREATMENT	CO, CT, IA, MI
CLASSIFY HIV AS AN STD	AL, FL, IL, KY, MS, MT, NV, SC, TN, UT, VT, WY
CLASSIFY HIV AS A COMMUNICABLE, CONTAGIOUS, OR INFECTIOUS DISEASE	AL, ID, MT, NC, OK, TX, VA
PERMIT MINORS TO CONSENT TO DIAGNOSIS AND TREATMENT OF REPORTABLE DISEASES	CA, PA
SPECIFIC EMANCIPATION OR MATURE MINOR STATUTES	AL, AK, AZ, CA, CO, GA, IL, IN, KY, LA, MA, MD, MN, MS, MO, MT, NV, NM, NY, OK, PA, RI, SC, TX, VA, WY

An Oregon study (CDC, 1992) found that adolescents were more likely to seek HIV testing at private sector test sites than publicly funded sites. This preference was not explained. An examination of homeless and runaway youth found that younger adolescents were more likely to be tested at private physicians' offices or hospitals than publicly funded testing sites (Goodman & Berecochea, 1994). A Boston-based study of 9-12 graders found that the high school study group had a preference for interacting with physicians. The group reportedly felt comfortable with physicians and wanted physicians to initiate questions about HIV and HIV-related behaviors. No clear preference for a testing site was identified, but overall the group preferred to be tested by someone who did not know them, especially the female students (Rawitscher, Saitz & Freidman, 1995). These studies may indicate that younger adolescents, especially minors, prefer to seek out some form of physician assistance in the HIV testing process. It may be a verbal exchange of information or the actual testing itself, but physicians play a key role. The concern to remain anonymous is an important one as well.

In the state of Colorado, where minors are allowed to consent to HIV testing, a study of youth (average age 15 years) seeking testing and those not seeking testing found results which support the argument that adolescents who seek out HIV testing are at greater risk o infection than those who do not (Main, Iverson & McGloin, 1994) The adolescents who were tested were more than twice as likely t(have had sexual intercourse with a greater number of partners at ; younger age, and more than three times as likely to have injecte(drugs.

As with HIV prevention education services, perhaps the best envi ronment in which minors may access HIV testing is the school School-based HIV testing programs reduce many of the barriers mi nors may face such as access, knowledge of a testing site, and finan cial burden. In 1995, *AIDS Policy and Law* (1995) reported that th(longest-running school-based HIV testing program had come to a1 end due to the objections of parents. For three years, the Florid; program provided free voluntary testing. Students did need writte1 permission from parents to be tested, but the results remained confi dential, which may be why students chose to use the school-base(program. Program supporters and educators felt the program was ; success as the number of adolescents testing positive for HIV droppe(over the three years, as students became more aware of the behavior that put them at risk.

National data from the CDC indicates that adolescents (age 13-19 are utilizing HIV counseling and testing services in a limited fashio1 (Rotheram-Borus et al., 1997). National studies have also found tha those adolescents seeking HIV counseling and testing services at pub licly funded sites had below average post-test return rates (Valdiserr et al., 1993). Little is known about what influences an adolescent' decision to be tested. In adults, testing behaviors may be related t(identification of symptoms or the acknowledgment of risk-taking be haviors. Many adolescents live at home with family members and ma' experience barriers to accessing HIV counseling and testing services Some minors may not be clear as to their rights to consent to testing, o where to go to be tested. Confidentiality may also be a barrier t(testing for some minors. The predominant modes of HIV transmissio1 in adolescents–unprotected sexual intercourse and injection dru{ use–are sensitive issues to discuss with parents. Requesting consen for an HIV test may mean an admittance of sexual activity or drug use When a legislative change in the state of Connecticut granted minor the right to consent to testing, the numbers of minors tested for HI\ increased twofold (Meehan, Hansen & Klein, 1997).

TREATMENT

In many states, if a minor may consent to be tested for a certain disease, the minor may also consent to the treatment of such a disease (AMA, 1993). As discussed earlier, statutes exist in all states allowing minors to consent to STD diagnosis and treatment. This came about as a result of the epidemic of STDs in teenagers. The ability of minors to consent to HIV treatment is a bit less clear.

Relatively speaking, HIV and AIDS are new diseases. The science and treatment of HIV infection and AIDS have changed considerably since the epidemic was first identified. Progressive research has allowed the treatment of HIV infection to develop from single-drug therapy that loses impact over time, to multiple high-potency drug regimes that attack the replication of the virus at many levels. Unfortunately, minors have not always been included in the research that has led to such life-sustaining treatments.

Before a new pharmacologic agent can receive approval for HIV-related treatment for humans, it must pass through three phases of clinical trials to determine the efficacy of the drug. Clinical trials for HIV treatments are funded by the Federal Drug Administration (FDA), the National Institutes of Health (NIH), and the National Institute of Allergy and Infectious Diseases (NIAID) (D'Angelo, 1992; Hengeller et al., 1992). Prior to 1989, protocols for drug trials had been approved only for adults aged 18 years or older, or for children from birth to 13 years of age. Adolescents aged 13-17 years were initially completely excluded. In 1989, 13-17 year olds were allowed to become part of the Pediatric Clinical Trials Group. In 1992, a congressional mandate prompted the establishment of programs specifically aimed at recruiting adolescents for clinical trials (D'Angelo, 1992). Today, the age protocol has been expanded for many clinical trials for HIV treatment to include ages 0-99 years, or 13-99 years. Of the 156 open clinical trials identified as of October 1997, 86 have protocols allowing 13-17 year olds to enroll in the trial (personal communication, Clinical Trials Information Service, CDC, 24 October 1997).

Treatment recommendations for the care of adolescents with HIV infection and AIDS have been documented (Futterman & Hein, 1992; Society for Adolescent Medicine, 1993). Researchers believe, however, that the number of adolescents receiving care is far lower than those who are actually infected with HIV (DiLorenzo et al., 1993). This may be due to a lack of age-specific services for adolescents, lack of knowledge of services, or fear of disclosure of their HIV status. *A* study conducted with the first 50 patients of the Adolescent AIDS Program at the Montefiore Medical Center, Bronx, New York, found that consequences of disclosing HIV infection were an overwhelming issue for all patients (Futterman et al., 1993). Several of the adolescents studied were forced to leave their homes or their foster home once they disclosed their status. Many feared they would be forced to leave school and were reluctant to take medication out of fear it would reveal their HIV status.

There are currently four states with specific legislation which allows minors to consent to HIV treatment (English, 1992). In the state of Connecticut, a minor may consent to treatment of HIV without parental/guardian notification if that notification would potentially jeopardize the treatment (Connecticut General Statutes § 19a-581 592). Even in the absence of statues, courts have been willing to apply the "mature" minor and "emancipated" minor doctrines and thus protect the provider from liability from providing treatment (English 1990). There have been no reported decisions in which a provider has been sued for providing non-negligent care to a minor without the consent of a parent or guardian (AMA, 1993). Empirical studies have provided little support for the assumption that minors, especially those aged 14 years and older, lack the capacity to make rational health care decisions (Weithorn & Campbell, 1982; Lewis, 1981; Kaser-Boyd et al., 1985).

Providing treatment to adolescents, especially minors, raises issues that are not generally raised when dealing with younger children (Sikand, Schubiner & Simpson, 1997). Adolescence is a time of cognitive, physiologic, psychological and psychosocial change. These changes vary greatly with each adolescent and in turn, affect the adolescent's ability to understand treatment and make treatment decisions. The treatment of HIV infection and AIDS is very complex. The changing nature of the disease, the frequency of viral load tests and CD4 counts, and the complex treatment regimes being advocated by the National Institutes of Health (1997) make treatment a complicated undertaking. This is not to overlook the psychosocial aspects of infection. They are complicated and complex, and much less well studied in the adolescent population than the adult population.

DISCUSSION

Minors represent a distinct segment of the population. They face a struggle between childhood and adulthood. This struggle is social, psychological, physiological and legal. The introduction of HIV into the minor and adolescent populations has only served to magnify this struggle. How society views minors impacts public policy. Public policy impacts minors' ability to receive services that relate to HIV infection. Early policy concerning AIDS was driven by defined "risk groups" in which adolescents were not included. Today, many polices and funding sources are linked to "case counting," which still leaves adolescents marginalized as reported AIDS cases in the 13-19 year age category represent .48% of all reported cases (CDC, 1997). It is important to restate, however, that of the 29 states which mandate the reporting of HIV infection, 3,574 cases of HIV infection have been reported in the adolescent age category. This figure is greater than the number of reported cases of AIDS, which is reported in every state, and it only represents a little over half of the nation. The adolescent population cannot wait until AIDS case reporting and HIV reporting have reached high enough figures to be recognized by the federal government.

It is clear that minors engage in behaviors that put them at risk for HIV infection. It becomes clear, then, that minors should have the right to access and consent to services reflective of these behaviors. Risk behaviors most likely do not vary across state lines as do the laws governing who may consent to receive services related to these behaviors. D'Angelo (1992) calls for all states to recognize HIV infection as an STD. If HIV were nationally defined as an STD, minors would be able to consent to testing and treatment based on existing STD statutes. Unless there is intense pressure from the federal government, this is unlikely to happen, as local legislation is generally left to the discretion of the states.

The removal of legal barriers to HIV services does not necessarily remove the non-legal barriers for minors. Although it has been documented that school-based condom availability programs do not increase rates of sexual activity but increase condom use (Guttmacher et al., 1997), condom availability programs do not exist in all school systems. They are completely absent from some states altogether (personal communication, S. Alford, Advocates For Youth, 2 October 1997). Some minors may not be able to purchase condoms due to lack of finances or due to the social burden of purchasing them in a publi place.

In many states minors may have legal access to HIV counseling an testing services. They may not, however, know where the sites ar located, feel comfortable at certain site locations or have adequat transportation. The non-legal barriers to receiving treatment for HI' infection are more complex. Many minors lack knowledge of th availability of medical services, and lack health insurance (Dougherty 1993). The availability of age-specific treatment providers is lackin as well. These factors are magnified for minors who live in non-metro politan areas.

The public health profession needs to continue to examine th unique legal position of the minor population, but at the same tim cannot overlook the non-legal barriers to HIV services. A comprehen sive and accessible continuum of care that ranges from prevention t treatment is the only way to prevent, identify, and treat infectior Without well-established linkages between different levels of service and care, minors will be lost in a fragmented system. The importanc of prevention efforts cannot be stated enough. It is estimated tha 40,000 new cases of HIV infection occur in the U.S. each year and a many as 25% may be among young people under the age of 22 (CDC 1998). Surveys suggest that prevention messages have helped to in crease the amount of condom use among adolescents who are sexuall active, but have not increased the amount of sexual activity (CDC 1998). Five-year trends from the Youth Risk Behavior Survey (YRBS suggest that more must be done to educate adolescents on the delay o the initiation of sexual activity and the reduction in risky sexual be havior (CDC, 1998). Prevention programs must be comprehensive an originate from a variety of sources. School-based programs are no enough and do not reach all adolescents. The inclusion of primary car physicians in HIV prevention education is crucial. Studies have show1 that primary care physicians do not always educate their adolescen patients about STD/HIV transmission, and screen for sexual activit and provide condoms on an less regular basis (Millstein, Igra & Gans 1996). If adolescents receive prevention messages from a variety o sources, the more likely they are to "hear" the messages and actuall initiate safer behavior.

Today's minors represent the first generation born into the HI\ epidemic. This generation does not know life without HIV or AIDS

Hein (1992) suggests that "the social and economic well-being of this first 'AIDS generation' may well predict the future well-being of this nation as a whole in the next century" (page 3). This first "AIDS generation" should have the legal right to access HIV services and care. Future generations depend on it.

REFERENCES

American Medical Association (AMA) Council on Scientific Affairs. Confidential Health Services for Adolescents. *Journal of the American Medical Association*, 1993. 269. 1420-1423.

Annas G. *Standard of Care The Law of American Bioethics*. New York: Oxford University Press. 1993.

Briefs. *AIDS Policy & Law*, 1995. 10. p. 2.

Brown BR, Baranowshi MD, Kulig JW, Stephenson JN et al. Searching For The Magic Johnson Effect: AIDS, Adolescence and Celebrity Disclosure. *Adolescence*, 1996. 31. 253-264.

Canterbury RJ, McGarvey EL, Sheldon-Keller AE et al. Prevalence of HIV-Related Risk Behaviors and STDs Among Incarcerated Adolescents. *Journal of Adolescent Health*, 1995. 17. 173-177.

Centers for Disease Control and Prevention (CDC). Adolescents and HIV/AIDS. March 1998.

Centers for Disease Control and Prevention (CDC). Facts About Condoms and Their Use in Preventing HIV Infection and Other STDs. *HIV/AIDS Prevention*, July 30, 1993a.

Centers for Disease Control and Prevention (CDC). *HIV/AIDS Surveillance Report*, 1994. 6. 2. p. 16.

Centers for Disease Control and Prevention (CDC). *HIV/AIDS Surveillance Report*, 1995. 7. 2. p. 14.

Centers for Disease Control and Prevention (CDC). *HIV/AIDS Surveillance Report*, 1996. 8. 2. pgs . 15, 16, 34.

Centers for Disease Control and Prevention (CDC). *HIV/AIDS Surveillance Report*, 1997. 9. 2. pgs . 15, 16, 37.

Centers for Disease Control and Prevention (CDC). Sexual Behaviors of STD Clinic Patients Before and After Earvin "Magic" Johnson's HIV-Infection Announcement–Maryland, 1991-92. *Journal of the American Medical Association*, 1993b. 269. 977-978.

Centers for Disease Control and Prevention. Testing for HIV in the Public and Private Sectors–Oregon, 1988-1991. *Morbidity and Mortality Weekly Report*, 1992. 41. 581-584.

D'Angelo LJ, Getson PR, Luban NLC & Gayle HD. Human Immunodeficiency Virus Infection in Urban Adolescents: Can We Predict Who is at Risk? *Pediatrics*, 1991. 88. 982-986.

D'Angelo LJ. Public Policy HIV Disease and Adolescents. In R. DiClemente (Ed).

Adolescents and AIDS: A Generation in Jeopardy (p 249-261). Newbury Park Sage Publications. 1992.

DiLorenzo TA, Abramo DM, Hein K et al. The Evaluation of Targeted Outreach in an Adolescent HIV/AIDS Program. *Journal of Adolescent Health*, 1993. 13 301-306.

Dougherty DM. Adolescent Health: Reflection on a Report to the US Congress *American Psychologist*, 1993. 48. 193-201.

English A. AIDS Testing and Epidemiology for Youth. Recommendations of the Work Group. *Journal of Adolescent Health Care*, 1989. 10. 52s-57s.

English A. Expanding Legal Access to HIV Services for Adolescents: Legal and Ethical Issues. In R. DiClemente (Ed). *Adolescents and AIDS: A Generation in Jeopardy* (p. 262-283). Newbury Park: Sage Publications. 1992.

English A. Runaway and Street Youth at Risk for HIV Infection: Legal and Ethical Issues in Access to Care. *Journal of Adolescent Health*, 1991. 12. 504-510.

English A. Treating Adolescents, Legal and Ethical Considerations. *Medical Clinics of North America*, 1990. 74. 1097-1112.

Futtterman D & Hein K. Care of HIV-Infected Adolescents. *AIDS Clinical Care*, 1992. 4. 95-98.

Futterman D, Hein K, Reuben N et al. Human Immunodeficiency Virus-Infected Adolescents: the First 50 Patients in a New York City Program. *Pediatrics*, 1993 91. 730-735.

Futterman D, Hein K & Kunins H. Teens and AIDS Identifying and Testing Those at Risk. *Contemporary Pediatrics*, 1993. 68-93.

Gittler J, Quigley-Rich M & Saks MJ. *Adolescents' Health Care Decision Making: The Law and Public Policy*. New York: Carnegie Council on Adolescent Development. 1990.

Goodman E & Berecochea JE. Predictors of HIV Testing Among Runaway and Homeless Adolescents. *Journal of Adolescent Health*, 1994. 15. 566-572.

Grubman S, Gross E, Lerner-Weiss N et al. Older Children and Adolescents Living with Perinatally Acquired Human Immunodeficiency Virus. *Pediatrics*, 1995. 95. 657-663.

Guttmacher S, Lieberman L, Ward D et al. Condom Availability in New York City Public High Schools: Relationships to Condom Use and Behavior. *American Journal of Public Health*, 1997. 87. 1427-1433.

Guttmacher SG, Lieberman L, Ward D et al. Parents' Attitudes and Beliefs About HIV/AIDS Prevention with Condom Availability in New York City Public High Schools. *Journal of School Health*, 1995. 65. 101-106.

Hein K. Adolescents at Risk for HIV Infection. In R. DiClemente (Ed). *Adolescents and AIDS: A Generation in Jeopardy*, (p. 3-16). Newbury Park: Sage Publications. 1992.

Henggeler SW, Melton GB & Rodrigue JR. *Pediatric and Adolescent AIDS Research Findings from the Social Sciences*. Newbury Park: Sage Publications. 1992.

Hofstetter CR, Horell MF, Myers CA et al. Patterns of Communication About AIDS among Hispanic and Anglo Adolescents. *American Journal of Preventive Medicine*, 1995. 11. 231-237.

Holder AR. Disclosure and Consent in Pediatrics. *Law Medicine and Health Care*, 1988. 16. 219-228.

Holder A. *Legal Issues in Pediatrics and Adolescent Medicine*. New York: John Wiley & Sons. 1977.

Holder AR. Minors' Rights to Consent to Medical Care. *Journal of the American Medical Association*, 1987. 257. 3400-3402.

Holtzman D, Andersen JE, Kann L et al., HIV Instruction, HIV Knowledge and Drug Injection Among High School Students in the United States. *American Journal of Public Health*, 1991. 81. 1596-1601.

Hou SI & Basen-Engquist K. Human Immunodeficiency Virus Risk Behavior Among Asian/Pacific Islander High School Students in the United States: Does Culture Make a Difference? *Journal of Adolescent Health*, 1997. 20:1. 68-74.

Intergovernmental Health Policy Project (IHPP) George Washington University. States that Specifically Allow Minors to Consent to HIV/STD Testing. Unpublished document. 1994.

Kaser-Boyd N, Adelman HS, Taylor L & Perry N. Minors Ability to Identify Risks and Benefits of Therapy. *Professional Psychology: Research & Practice*, 1985. 16. 411-417.

Keller SE, Bartlett JA, Schleifer SJ et al., HIV-Relevant Sexual Behavior Among a Healthy Inner-City Heterosexual Adolescent Population in an Endemic Area of HIV. *Journal of Adolescent Health*, 1991. 12. 44-48.

Kirby D. School-Based Prevention Programs: Design, Evaluation and Effectiveness. In R. DiClemente (Ed). *Adolescents and AIDS: A Generation in Jeopardy* (p. 159-180). Newbury Park: Sage Publications. 1992

Leo J, Delany P & Whitaker L. Sex and Schools. *Time*, November 1986.

Lewis CC. How Adolescents Approach Decisions: Changes Over Grades Seven to Twelve and Policy Implications. *Child Development*, 1981. 52. 538-544.

Main DS, Iverson DC & McGloin J. Comparison of HIV-Risk Behaviors and Demographics of Adolescents Tested or Not Tested for HIV Infection. *Public Health Reports*, 1994. 109. 600-702.

Marsiglio W & Mott F. The Impact of Sex Education Sexual Activity Contraceptive Use and Premarital Pregnancy among American Teenagers. *Family Planning Perspectives*, 1986. 18. 151-162.

Meehan TM, Hansen H & Klein W. The Impact of Parental Consent on the HIV Testing of Minors. *American Journal of Public Health*, 1997. 87. 1338-1341.

Miller SG, Igra V & Gans J. Delivery of STD/HIV Preventive Services to Adolescents by Primary Care Physicians. *Journal of Adolescent Health*, 1996. 19:4. 249-257.

National Abortion and Reproductive Rights Action League (NARAL). Sex Education in America: A State by State Review, 1995.

National Institutes of Health (NIH). *Guidelines For the Use of Antiretroviral Agents in HIV-Infected Adults and Adolescents*. Draft. June 1997.

Norman J & Harris M. *The Private Life of the American Teenager*. New York: Rawson Wade. 1981.

North RL. Legal Authority for HIV Testing of Adolescents. *Journal of Adolescent Health*, 1990. 11. 176-187.

Plotkin R. When Rights Collide: Parents, Children and Consent to Treatment. *Jour nal of Pediatric Psychology*, 1981. 6. 121-130.

Ratwitscher LA, Saitz R & Freidman LS. Adolescents' Preferences Regarding Hu man Immunodeficiency Virus (HIV)-Related Physician Counseling and HIV Testing. *Pediatrics*, 1995. 96. 52-58.

Rosenberg PS, Biggar RJ & Goedert JJ. Declining Age at HIV Infection in the United States. *New England Journal of Medicine*, 1994. 330. 789 (letter).

Rotheram-Borus MJ, Gillis JR, Reid HM et al., HIV Testing, Behaviors, and Knowl edge Among Adolescents at High Risk. *Journal of Adolescent Health*, 1997. 20 216-225.

Sigman GS & O'Conner C. Explorations for Physicians of the Mature Minor Doc trine. *Journal of Pediatrics*, 1991. 119. 520-525.

Sikand A, Schubiner H & Simpson PM. Parent and Adolescent Perceived Need fo Parental Consent Involving Research with Minors. *Archives of Pediatric an Adolescent Medicine*, 1997. 151. 603-607.

Society for Adolescent Medicine. HIV/AIDS Medical Management. *Journal of Ado lescent Health*, 1993. 14. 36s-52s.

Stiffman AR, Cunningham R & Dore P. Magic Johnson. *Journal of Adolescen Health*, 1993. 14. 427 (letter).

Valdiserri RO, Moore M, Gerber AR et al., A Study of Clients Returning for Coun seling After HIV Testing: Implications for Improving Rates of Return. *Public Health Reports,* 1993. 108. 12-18.

Vermund SH, Hein K Gayle HD et al., Acquired Immunodeficiency Syndrome Among Adolescents, Case Surveillance Profiles in New York City and the Rest o the United States. *American Journal of Disease in Children*, 1989. 143 1220-1224.

Walter HJ, Vaughan RD, Gladis MM et al., Factors Associated with AIDS Risk Behaviors Among High School Students in an AIDS Epicenter. *American Journa of Public Health*, 1992. 82. 528-532.

Weithorn LA & Campbell SB. The Competency of Children and Adolescents to Make Informed Treatment Decisions. *Child Development*, 1982. 53. 1589-1598.

Wing K. *The Law and the Public's Health*. Michigan: Health Administration Press 1990.

In the Best Interest of the Child: Maintaining Family Integrity Among HIV-Positive Mothers, Children, and Adolescents

Dorie J. Gilbert

SUMMARY. Women are increasingly represented among cases of acquired immunodeficiency syndrome (AIDS) and acquired human immunodeficiency virus (HIV) infection. This article discusses challenges faced by HIV-positive mothers in parenting their children and adolescents, challenges which may increase their involvement with child welfare, school, legal, and community services prior to guardianship needs. The article then addresses the heightened importance that parenting takes on for many HIV-positive mothers and discusses how preserving the parent-child bond can be pivotal in acting in the best interest of the child. *[Article copies available for a fee from The Haworth Document Delivery Service: 1-800-342-9678. E-mail address: getinfo@haworthpressinc.com]*

KEYWORDS. HIV, AIDS, HIV-positive mothers, parenting concerns

Approximately three-quarters of HIV-positive women have children (Niebuhr, Hughes, & Pollard, 1994). As mothers of young children and adolescents, HIV-positive mothers are faced with the dual

Dorie J. Gilbert, PhD, is Assistant Professor, The University of Texas at Austin, School of Social Work, 1925 San Jacinto Boulevard, Suite 3.130M, Austin, TX 78712.

[Haworth co-indexing entry note]: "In the Best Interest of the Child: Maintaining Family Integrity Among HIV-Positive Mothers, Children, and Adolescents." Gilbert, Dorie J. Co-published simultaneously in *Journal of HIV/AIDS Prevention & Education for Adolescents & Children* (The Haworth Press, Inc.) Vol. 3, No. 1/2, 1999, pp. 99-117; and: *HIV Affected and Vulnerable Youth: Prevention Issues and Approaches* (ed: Susan Taylor-Brown and Alejandro Garcia) The Haworth Press, Inc., 1999, pp. 99-117. Single or multiple copies of this article are available for a fee from The Haworth Document Delivery Service [1-800-342-9678, 9:00 a.m. - 5:00 p.m. (EST). E-mail address: getinfo@haworthpressinc.com].

© 1999 by The Haworth Press, Inc. All rights reserved.

challenge of managing their illness while maintaining their parentin role to HIV-infected or HIV-affected children. For many women, th parent-child bond takes on renewed importance in the midst of suffei ing and loss. Women living with HIV or AIDS are usually the sol supporter of themselves and their children (Barlow, 1992; Schable (al., 1995). For most of these women and children, AIDS is entrenche within the larger societal woes of socioeconomic deprivation (Farme 1996). In such cases, AIDS becomes simply another of the tragedie associated with severely impoverished living: inadequate housin; poor health, violence, isolation, discrimination, and substance abus (Conners, 1996). Not surprisingly, many of the variables associate with AIDS among women and children similarly describe the familie who are most often in need of an array of child welfare and othe social services.

A number of articles have addressed the increased involvement c child welfare agencies in finding substitute placements for the alarn ing number of children orphaned due to their parents' death or in paired abilities from AIDS (Carten & Fennoy, 1997; Cohen & Net ring, 1994; Taylor-Brown, 1991). However, given the time betwee HIV infection and progression to AIDS, many HIV-positive mother may become involved with various institutions long before guardiar ship needs arise. For example, women and their children may come t the attention of child welfare, mental health, school, juvenile justic and legal systems because of inadequate housing and other unfulfille basic needs, a child's health and educational concerns, or parentin difficulties precipitated by a child's reactions to HIV-related stress.

Yet, the pervasive stigma associated with AIDS persists in increas ing HIV-positive mothers' tendencies towards self-blame, shame, fea of disclosure, and hesitancy to access child welfare and other service: During the first decade of the pandemic, Miller and Carlton (1988 suggested that vertical (mother-to-fetus) transmission of HIV be ir cluded in definitions of child abuse and neglect. While this policy ha never been widely espoused, HIV-positive women are likely to pei ceive themselves as vulnerable targets of social service agencies. In recent study, researchers noted that women often feared "they coul lose their children if others became aware of their status" (Hack Somlai, Kelly, & Kalichman, 1997, p. 54). These perceptions high light the need for professionals to understand the unique meaning tha parenting and family takes on for HIV-positive mothers.

Children living with an HIV-positive mother comprise the largest group of AIDS-affected biologic families (Fair, Spencer, Wiener, & Riekert, 1995). However, HIV-infected or affected children may reside with foster parents, extended family, and non-blood relatives. In some cases, HIV-infected and affected children live with a biological father, who may or may not be HIV-positive. While HIV-affected families of any configuration will face parenting and bonding concerns, this paper focuses on the experiences of HIV-positive, biological mothers, many of whom are in single-parent situations, in some cases due to the death of a husband or male partner from AIDS. The author discusses challenges faced by HIV-positive mothers in parenting their children and adolescents, challenges which may increase their involvement with child welfare and other community agencies prior to guardianship needs. The article then addresses the heightened importance that parenting takes on for many HIV-positive mothers. As a result, preserving the parent-child bond can be pivotal in acting in the best interest of the child. A case study is presented to further clarify how maintaining the mother-child bond in the face of impending mortality becomes crucial in assisting HIV-positive women to safeguard not only their children's well-being but their own human dignity.

HIV-POSITIVE WOMEN AND THEIR CHILDREN

The AIDS pandemic has affected millions globally and, within the United States, the disease that was first publicized as a gay-male plague has now spread substantially beyond this group. Although males, primarily gay and bisexual males, still account for the majority of cases, women are increasingly represented among cases of AIDS and HIV infection, with AIDS cases among women rising from 7% in 1985 to 20% in 1997 (Centers for Disease Control [CDC] Surveillance Report, June 1997). Moreover, the majority of HIV-positive women are of childbearing age and approximately 7000 of these women give birth to infants annually (HIV Survey in Childbearing, 1996). While early reports on HIV-infected females emphasized women's intravenous (IV) drug-using as the major mode of transmission, the percentage of women infected through heterosexual contact with an HIV-infected person (39%) is nearly as high as the rate of infection due to a woman's history of IV drug use (44%) according to recent trends (CDC, 1997).

Women's experiences with HIV infection are affected by both thei inferior status and absent or misdirected public policy toward womei and minorities (Kaplan, 1995; Land, 1994; Lea, 1994; Wilton, 1997) Land (1994, p. 355) notes that "society's blatant neglect of disease prevention practices, and the United States' institutionalized prejudic against women and people of color have served to create an invisibl but continuously growing population of HIV-infected women of col or." Thus, African American and Hispanic women have been dispro portionately affected, representing over three-fourths of cases reportec among women, although these two groups combined only comprise 21% of the U.S. population. While a heterogeneous group, Africai American and Hispanic women share a history of being racially disen franchised, economically oppressed, and socially disadvantaged. Sub sequently, relative risks for AIDS associated with IV drug use anc poverty are much higher for ethnic-minority than·for white popula tions (Singer, 1992). Mirroring the racial distribution among women African American and Hispanic children account for 81% of reportec AIDS cases among children (CDC, 1997).

The vast majority of HIV-infected children acquire the virus verti cally from their mothers. Although some HIV-infected children wil survive into late school-age and even early adolescence (Lewis, Hai ken, & Hoyt, 1994), about three-quarters of children will succumb tc the disease before the age of three years (Andiman, 1995). For adults the time between infection and the actual onset of AIDS extend nearly a decade for the majority of infected individuals (Smith & Moore, 1996), although some researchers have noted women to have ; shorter survival time than do men with AIDS (Lea, 1994; see Smith & Moore, 1996 for discussion of conflicting findings). Early detectioi and treatment prolong the asymptomatic stage for both adults anc children; however, even with improved treatment, HIV-positive moth ers will spend a number of years parenting and managing their HI\ infection while struggling with severe losses, stigma, and psychoso cial strain.

Of the scant literature addressing the needs of HIV-positive mother: and their children, the majority focuses on guardianship needs. Earl) projections of the number of AIDS orphans estimated that 82,000 tc 125,000 children would be orphaned due to AIDS by the year 200((Michaels & Levine, 1992). However, in recent years, HIV/AIDS rates among women have risen more rapidly than initially projected hus, there has been a continuing dramatic increase in the number of ɔrphaned young people. In the state of New York, 28,000 children and youth (to age 21) had been orphaned by maternal death from AIDS by the end of 1996; by the end of 2001, the number of AIDS orphans is ǝstimated at 58,000 for the state (Families in Crisis, 1997). Clearly, ʒuardianship needs must be addressed; yet, before children are actually orphaned or in need of substitute care, HIV-positive mothers and :heir children are often in need of concrete and psychosocial support from a range of social service agencies.

Most children born to HIV-infected mothers are living with a biological parent (55%) or with another relative (10%). Among women who are not drug-users, 78% of children live with a biological parent (Caldwell et al., 1992). Because children living with an HIV-positive mother comprise the largest group of children in AIDS-affected biological families (Fair et al., 1995), this article focuses on mother-child dyads, including both infected and healthy children. Healthy children in AIDS-affected families suffer as well. Non-infected children and adolescents are impacted by stigma, social isolation, and multiple losses, often in addition to the marginal living conditions predating the HIV infection. Because of the multiple losses experienced by healthy children, all children of HIV-positive parents may be considered at developmental risk (Brazdziunas, Roizen, Kohrman, & Smith, 1994). The parent-child dynamics of these families are described next.

HIV-POSITIVE MOTHERS' PARENTING CHALLENGES WITH CHILDREN AND ADOLESCENTS

Of children residing with an HIV-positive mother, no exact figures exist on how many are receiving in-home child welfare or other social services. Yet, it is evident that many of the same variables which place women and children at risk for HIV also increase the chance that a family will be involved with social services. HIV infection simply compounds that probability. An array of psychosocial stressors of family units coping with HIV/AIDS have been identified: adjusting to the diagnosis, dealing with how the infection was contracted, handling fears of contagion, coping with the fears and reality of social ostracism, redefining familial roles and responsibilities, preparing for the loss of the ill family member(s), and planning for the future (Tiblier, Walker, & Rolland, 1989). While parenting under normal circum-

stances can be described as difficult and demanding, it is under ex
tremely stressful conditions that HIV-positive mothers are parentin
their children and adolescents. The major challenges to parenting cor
cerns include: (1) the mother's general ability to provide for he
children, including the special medical needs of infected childrei
and (2) managing the emotional well-being of affected children an
adolescents.

Mother's General Ability to Provide for Her Children

Given a lower economic status, many mothers living with HIV
AIDS may have difficulties providing for their children. Financial an
housing concerns rank high among women living with HIV/AID!
(Gillman & Newman, 1996). Women's struggles with finances an
lack of adequate housing place them in a high probability of bein
identified by child protective workers in the area of neglect. In a stud
exploring stress and coping in families affected by pediatric AID!
Mellins and Ehrhardt (1994) found that compared to uninfected care
givers, HIV-infected parents reported more isolation and fewer finar
cial and support resources. Recent multistate survey results indicat
that 85% of HIV-infected mothers were not working and 72% ha
incomes less than $10,000 (Schable et al., 1995), thus, the majorit
may be receiving AFDC or some other form of public assistance. Ye
women may be either unaware of or hesitant to use AIDS-relate
resources due to shame and secrecy and because of fear of bein
identified as neglectful mothers. Mothers are also subject to havin
AFDC benefits cut if children are removed from their care. Moreove
because women may not be aware of housing and other benefits avail
able to HIV-positive individuals, many HIV-infected women will nc
have access to needed services.

Drug-using, HIV-positive mothers are those most likely to be in
volved with child protection services. The increase in substance abus
problems, including the crack-cocaine epidemic, has greatly increase
the number of children in out-of-home care. Termed the twin epidem
ics, substance abuse can be considered a dual epidemic with HI'
disease (Dansky, 1997; Groze, Haines-Simeon, & Barth, 1994). Th
literature notes several reasons for the increased representation i
foster care of children born to drug-using, HIV-positive women. On
reason is that women who use drugs may be perceived as unable t
care properly for their children. Also, drug-using mothers are mor

likely than non-drug using HIV-positive women to come to the attention of child protective services due to aggressive referral systems among health care providers (Caldwell, Thomas, & Parrott, 1992). However, when these mothers are cooperative and capable of accessing services, they may have difficulties finding programs that accept mother-children dyads or even provide childcare (Taylor-Brown, 1993). Drug-using women may have the fewest financial resources and may be cut off from family support due to previous drug use, making their parenting even more difficult to accomplish.

HIV-positive mothers may also be caring for an HIV-infected child. In addition to eventual physical deterioration, children with HIV infection may present with various neurological and developmental problems, growth delays, and speech, motor, and cognitive regressions. Accessing and utilizing the necessary social services to address the child's many medical needs may be extremely difficult for some mothers. Findings from one study indicate that children and caregivers' HIV status, additional or unusual caregiving demands, and a child's developmental delay status significantly influence parents' perceived stress (Lesar, Gerner, & Semmel, 1995). Unfortunately, a mother's inability to deal openly with her own status may translate into neglect in terms of failing to obtain needed medical care for herself as well as for an HIV-infected child.

HIV-positive mothers may become emotionally strained by their condition. Feelings of grief and loss are extensive, particularly when an HIV-positive mother is mourning the death of a child or partner to AIDS, while continuing her caretaker role for children. HIV-positive mothers are especially plagued with self-blame and self-hatred; the guilt associated with either having passed on a fatal disease to their children or leaving behind uninfected children can become overwhelming (Land, 1994). In one study, self-blame or attributing the cause of the HIV status to self was significantly positively correlated with depression, anxiety, and negative mood (Commerford et al., 1994). Women who lack necessary social support from family because they must keep their HIV status a secret carry an enormous burden. The children also bear this burden.

Emotional Well-Being of Affected Children and Adolescents

When HIV/AIDS is involved, psychoemotional risks associated with parenting are high for both parent and children. Reactions to

HIV/AIDS within the family can result in realignment of roles be
tween parents and children (Fair et al., 1995; Lewis, 1995). Childre
who must take on the role of caretaking for an ill parent or sibling ma
feel they are being unfairly burdened or punished, particularly whe
the added responsibilities are not developmentally appropriate (And
man, 1995; Fair et al., 1995). The stress experienced by uninfecte
children may result in lower grades and problems in school (Fanos &
Wiener, 1994). Healthy children may also have limits imposed on the
activities and interactions with peers (Andiman, 1995), which, in turr
may lead children to withdraw socially at school and within the
immediate community. In interviews with HIV-positive mother:
Faithful (1997) found that, in an attempt to avoid being harsh c
punitive, mothers may be too lenient, sometimes to the point of caus
ing children to act out or experience disciplinary problems.

Parent-adolescent relationships may be particularly strained. Teer
agers may have a number of developmentally-related barriers to cop
ing with a parent's HIV-positive status and illness. First, teenager
may perceive any additional responsibilities at home to be a threat t
new independence and autonomy (Fair et al., 1995). In addition, th
strong need for peer group approval may increase the adolescent's fea
of rejection from peers when and if a disclosure is made. Moreove
the egocentricism experienced during adolescence may impede th
ability of teenagers to empathize with parents and to see past their ow
needs at this stage.

Several authors have reported on conduct problems among adoles
cent children of parents with AIDS. Draimin (1993) interviewed 4
families with adolescent children, half of whom had already experi
enced a parent's death. Among this group of adolescents, a larg
number (73%) were experiencing problems at school and another 34%
were acting out at home. Rotheram and colleagues (as cited in Gardne
& Preator, 1996, p. 180) also found substantial problems among ado
lescents affected by parental AIDS, including skipping school (64%
and grade failure (56%). Lewis (1995) describes how an adolescent'
inability to cope with a parent's HIV infection can manifest in sever
behavioral and psychological problems, including destructive act:
suicidal ideation, uncontrolled defiance, and running away. Noting th
lack of controlled scientific research in this area, Lewis (1995) an
others raise caveats regarding assumptions of causality between HIV
AIDS and adolescents' behavioral problems. Rather, behavioral prob

lems of HIV-affected children and teens may not be substantially
higher than those experienced by non-HIV-affected children from similar backgrounds. Yet, the pervasive stigma and severe losses associated
with HIV along with repeated observations of such dynamics underscore the need to be aware of such potential secondary effects of HIV/
AIDS in parent-child dynamics.

Undoubtedly, HIV-positive mothers face many challenges in their
parenting role. Underlying their daily challenges is the pervasive stigma the family faces. For most HIV-positive mothers, this stigma is
compounded by societal sexism, racism, and classism–all of which
have impacted both the prevalence and perception of women living
with HIV and AIDS. One obvious strength of many HIV-positive
mothers is their perseverance in surviving life's adversities, the motivation for which is often inextricably tied to the mothering role.

THE HEIGHTENED IMPORTANCE
OF THE PARENT-CHILD BOND

Although HIV-positive women face many challenges as they manage the demands of their own illness while maintaining their role as
primary caretakers, relationships with children seem to provide the
thread that holds these women together. Faithfull (1997, p. 144) found
that for many HIV-positive women "children can offer the promise of
connection and the feeling of being needed and valued." Among
women in Gillman and Newman's (1996) study, children provided
motivation for women to recover from drugs or to obtain decent housing to keep the family intact. In other interviews with women, Hackl et
al. (1997) reported that women focused mostly on maintaining a
happy environment for their children in spite of their own debilitating
illness. In working with HIV-positive women to create written legacies
for children and significant others, Gilbert (1997) also notes that children can become a catalyst for renewed growth and integrity among
mothers living with HIV. The mothers' actions tended to be guided by
a need to maintain a sense of parental status and dignity to protect
children's well-being. As posited by feminist theorists, the ethic of
caring and connectedness through relationships means that women
tend to place an enormous amount of importance on their relationships
with their children and intimate partners to maintain a sense of related-
ness. Lea (1994) adds that "caring may also be women's source of

personal integrity and strength if they judge their worth by their capac ity to care" (p. 494).

If they have dealt with a long history of adversities, HIV-positiv mothers may view their HIV-status as a "last chance," a time to focu on the most meaningful issues, which is often manifested in the re newed priority they give to the parenting role. Among drug-usin women, researchers found that concern for children acted as a promi nent motivator for women to end their addiction (Gillman & Newmar 1996). These same researchers reported that, among the HIV-positiv women interviewed, those with at least one child placed outside th home were more concerned about housing than were those with eithe no children or all their children living with them. Thus, children repre sent a reason to live, to go on, and to garner needed support an finances for necessary lifestyle changes. Because many women be came infected due to a underlying sense of powerlessness, low self-es teem, and social isolation, insight gained through their HIV diagnosi and impending mortality may be the first opportunity to reflect o their inner strengths. Women often become determined to overcom their weaknesses in order to give their best to themselves and thei children. In doing so, ironically, some women may ignore their HI status so that they may continue with the day-to-day activities c managing a household. This need to care may lead women to ignor their own health needs, resulting in a shortened survival time of livin with HIV/AIDS (Lea, 1994).

Lesar and Maldonado (1996) note that the most often reporte parental coping strategy among families of HIV-infected children wa focusing on strengthening the family life and maintaining a positiv outlook on life. Children suffering separation and loss from a parer are likely to experience long-term psychological consequences, ir cluding depression in adulthood (Bowlby, 1980). Logically, the quali ty of the parent-child bond and family connectedness will impac surviving children's responses to a parent's death. Although childre will naturally experience bereavement as they suffer the loss of moth ers, and in some instances, siblings and fathers, a strong parent-chil bond may buffer the long-lasting effects of parental loss on the chilc It is important that the children surviving their mothers emerge fror the crisis with a sense of emotional well-being. Resources, both con crete and therapeutic, are crucial to building on the natural strength c HIV-positive mothers in maintaining the health and well-being of th family. The following case study helps to illustrate the need for social service providers to consider parent-child bonding when working with HIV-positive mothers and their children.

CASE EXAMPLE

J is a 32-year-old Mexican-American mother of two boys, an 8-year-old and a 12-year-old, both healthy children. J discovered that she was HIV-positive two years ago and has continued to maintain her role as mother and caretaker to her children. However, the family was under increased stress due to conflicts between J and her adolescent son. After discovering that his mother was HIV-positive, the 12-year-old began experiencing difficulties at school and became disruptive at home. J took the initiative to consult with school officials regarding her son's reaction to her HIV-status but was unsuccessful in getting help from the school counselor. The 12-year-old eventually ran away and J became involved with child protective services for the first time when she solicited their help in finding her son. At that point, J's parenting ability became the target of the investigation, and she perceived that she was being unfairly targeted for investigations by child protective services. J was placed under investigation for parental neglect. J's 8-year-old son was immediately removed from the home and placed in temporary kinship care. Although J's extended family knew of her HIV-status, they generally displayed little empathy for those with HIV infection or AIDS. Thus, J was uncomfortable when visiting her son in the home of relatives. In the meantime, J discovered that her son had run away to live with his natural father, who also held strong prejudices against persons with HIV and AIDS. J felt that she had failed as a mother and these negative thoughts were being reinforced by her older son, ex-husband, and extended relatives. J became increasingly distraught over her separation from her youngest child and her older son's rejection of her due to her HIV status. Subsequently, J suffered an emotional breakdown. J feared she would die estranged from both her children.

The case was eventually dismissed following a six-month investigation. After obtaining needed counseling and support to work through issues of loss of dignity as a parent, J eventually returned home with her 8-year-old son. J consulted legal services to assist her in having her teenage son returned. The family is still in need of on-going counsel-

ing to help work through the stress both parent and children are expe
riencing as a result of family disruptions related to J's HIV-positiv
status and the initial lack of social service assistance.

THE CHALLENGE FOR SOCIAL SERVICE PROVIDERS

When parenting difficulties arise, HIV-positive mothers may com
in contact with a number of different institutions: the school system
juvenile justice system, and often child welfare services. The abov
case illustrates both challenges to and opportunities for service provi
sions with HIV-positive mothers and their children. Balancing th
competing interests of the child's safety and the preservation of th
family is especially crucial when families are also facing issues c
mortality and loss. Helping professionals are forced to deal with in
tensely personal and emotional issues of mothers who are strugglin,
to survive with HIV disease and are also experiencing parenting
financial, or other difficulties. Child welfare workers and other profes
sionals must operate with an adequate understanding of the dynamic
of women and children living with HIV infection. However, limita
tions faced by agencies, along with on-going fears, negative attitudes
and general reluctance of some to work directly with AIDS familie
create barriers to the provision of sensitive, effective intervention wit
HIV-positive mothers and their children.

Many HIV-positive mothers are likely to have some contact wit
child welfare agencies, whether through past, present or future cir
cumstances. In addition to the high turnover rates among child protec
tive service workers, low standards of many child welfare agencie
also diminish the effectiveness of working with HIV-positive mother
and their children. The concern for increased awareness on the part o
child protective service workers is heightened, given that few publi
child protective service workers have any formal training in socia
work. As discussed by Risley-Curtiss et al. (1997), most state welfar
agencies do not require entry-level workers to have completed bache
lor's or master's degrees in social work or related direct-service
experience. Disparities in ethnic characteristics of workers and client
also raise concerns. In essence, workers are predominantly youn;
Euro-Americans with limited social service experience or training
while the majority of HIV-positive mothers and children are African

American and Hispanic, usually struggling with a host of other problems in addition to HIV and AIDS.

Child welfare workers themselves have expressed concerns about their health safety when working closely with an HIV-infected client and may hold irrational fears or prejudices against persons with AIDS (Boland, Allen, Long, & Tasker, 1988). Such concerns are likely to persist despite increased knowledge about HIV and AIDS in recent years (Gillman, 1991). Social service providers, in general, may also hold negative beliefs about intravenous drug users and fears about working so closely with issues of death (Gillman, 1991).

Moreover, the emphasis on children has drawn attention away from the plight of mothers. In the early years of the epidemic, children with AIDS were afforded more sympathy and attention than their mothers in cases of vertical transmission. For almost a decade, women were part of an invisible epidemic (Corea, 1992, Patton 1994) and overlooked due to an overshadowing focus on infants and children with AIDS (Corea, 1992; Juhasz, 1990). Juhasz (1990) and Sacks (1996) suggest that an overplayed emphasis on the "innocent" child victims of AIDS served to further marginalize HIV-positive women as selfish procreators and blameworthy. Such perceptions of HIV-positive mothers may negatively impact the quality of services women receive. Workers may possess a strong sense of empathy for the child, but not see a need to engage the mother (Thompson, 1993). Barlow (1992) notes that the response from public human service departments is often focused on the removal or separation of the child from the mother or in some cases, so little assistance is afforded that mothers may relinquish their children. In addition, women who suffer overwhelming feelings of guilt and shame about passing the virus on to a child may succumb to thoughts of not deserving the child.

In addition to child welfare workers, those working within the school, juvenile, and legal systems are challenged to examine their own values and beliefs about AIDS and general feelings about individuals who are disenfranchised and lacking power in society. HIV-positive mothers are particularly vulnerable to rejection and loss of relationships (Corea, 1992). The fact that most women affected (i.e., women of color) have historically been disenfranchised and poverty-stricken also plays a role in their experiences with social service providers. Under ideal circumstances, HIV-positive parents should be treated with respect rather than punitively; the goal should be to build

on their parental strengths (Roberts, 1993; Thompson, 1993). Thu:
along with skills and knowledge in child development, family dynam
ics, children's rights, cultural differences, and other related areas, soci:
service workers need a clear understanding of the dynamics of HIV-al
fected families. Workers should be knowledgeable of HIV/AIDS liter:
ture and ways to coordinate health and human service systems in mee
ing the needs of families affected by the disease (Carten & Fenno:
1997). Furthermore, workers should have a clear understanding of hov
HIV-positive mothers have been objectified and labeled according t
risky behaviors, with little emphasis placed on their challenge to pare:
in the midst of stigma, grief, and impending mortality.

OPPORTUNITIES FOR INTERVENTION

In reviewing the case study, several opportunities for interventio
were present in J's case. The school system was the first to be con
tacted. School counselors are often in a position to help parents acce:
counseling and other resources. An initial school-based interventio
might have helped J access counseling and other services to addres
her older son's problems both at school and at home. HIV-affecte
children may display a number of emotional and behavioral response
to their stress and grief. Responses such as conduct problems or sud
den withdrawn behavior may first manifest at school. In some case:
children and adolescents may exhibit non-compliant and aggressiv
behavior that is symptomatic of anticipatory mourning, anger, an
anxiety about the impending loss of a loved one. Although juvenil
services were never involved in J's case, other adolescents from HIV
affected households may have an increased risk of juvenile delinquer
cy as they attempt to cope with their situation at home through runnin
away or disruptive behavior.

In cases where changing family dynamics have precipitated paren
child conflicts in AIDS-affected families, child welfare services ma
become involved. In J's case, a comprehensive, family-based assess
ment would have determined the nature and extent of services th
family needed. In the case study, there were ample opportunities fc
social service providers to build on J's existing parental strengths.
had taken the initiative to seek out family counseling. J had no pre
vious history of neglectful or abusive parenting. The most effectiv
intervention options would have involved maintaining the family:

integrity, providing in-home support services, and guiding J's attempts to obtain counseling and resources for her son. J placed a strong emphasis on her parental role. Her parenting attitude is reflected in her statement, "You try really hard to be a good parent. You want the time to be positive." In J's opinion, the assumption on the part of those from whom she sought help was "if she has HIV or AIDS, she must be on drugs or too sick to care for her children."

Finally, helping professionals must assess what role culture plays in any client's case. In J's case, exploring the importance of her Mexican-American heritage may have provided additional insight into her views on extended family, family orientation, social support networks and so on. Although J's extended family was supportive overall, their understanding of HIV and AIDS was limited. Culturally-sensitive, educational interventions could have enhanced the family's ability to support J and maintain good family relations.

CONCLUSION

The AIDS epidemic presents new and complex challenges to those who work to keep families together. One such challenge is to comprehend how AIDS has become a problem which both disintegrates family structures, yet acts to foster renewed family integrity and parent-child unity for many HIV-positive parents. The ever-increasing number of AIDS orphans draws attention not only to custody concerns but also to the need to preserve the well-being of parents and children in those years leading up to guardianship changes. Those directly involved with children and families are challenged to acknowledge the importance of the parent-child bond and the hope and motivation tied to a mother's desire to provide quality parenting in the face of uncertainty. The alarming increase in women identified as HIV-positive underscores the tragedy befalling mothers, children, and families, in general. Already facing extreme stigma and prejudices, HIV-positive mothers need to be assured that they will not be further stigmatized when involved with child welfare agencies, school systems, and juvenile justice or legal services. Most importantly, they need to be given every reasonable opportunity to maintain their dignity as parents as well as their ability to sustain their families.

Parenting challenges may result in HIV-positive mothers and children being involved with a number of agencies. When mothers experi-

ence difficulties in providing for their children, they may come unde
the scrutiny of child welfare agencies. When children experience emc
tional and conduct problems, fail to do well in school, or act out i
serious ways, school, juvenile justice, or other institutions will need t
interact with the family. Professionals must be prepared to address th
unique needs of these families in a sensitive manner.

On a broader level, society must act to help reduce the pervasiv
stigma associated with persons with HIV/AIDS. More programs ar
needed that assist HIV-positive mothers to disclose in a way tha
reduces risk of rejection but allows them to obtain necessary socia
services and social support. No doubt, prevention of HIV infection i
the ultimate goal and this is of particular concern for healthy childre
affected by AIDS. Children affected by their parent's HIV status hav
been noted to be at increased risk for HIV infection themselves due t
the severe losses and psychological trauma which may lead to thei
own risky behavior. Thus, the parent-child relationship is a crucia
focal point for prevention work.

Building positive relationships with HIV-positive mothers and chil
dren can assist the family in the long run. Once child welfare worker
recognize that they are working with an AIDS-affected family, the
will likely attempt to initiate guardianship discussions. Working wit
mothers around making appropriate plans for future custody of thei
children can present challenges. Nearly half of parents die before ther
are permanent guardianship plans for their children (Dansky, 1997
Many face emotional and practical barriers to making such decision
due to denial, secrecy, fear of isolation, lack of legal advice, difficult
in obtaining life insurance, fear of disclosing a current or previou
substance abuse problem, and lack of trust in child welfare or othe
service providers. If women have had negative experiences with chil
welfare and other agencies in the past, they are unlikely to seek hel
from traditional institutions that have historically failed to meet the
needs. Strong supports are needed for policies, programs and practice
which recognize the central importance of parenting and maintainin
parent-child bonds with HIV-positive mothers and their children. A
part of their parenting role, HIV-positive mothers will need to prepar
their children for a motherless future. Programs which allow mother
to act with integrity and to play an active role in planning for thei
children have the best chance of meeting the family's needs in
holistic manner.

REFERENCES

Andiman, W. (1995). Medical aspects of AIDS: What do children witness? In S. Geballe, J. Gruendel, & W. Andiman (Eds.), *Forgotten children of the AIDS epidemic* (pp. 32-49). New Haven, CT: Yale University Press.

Barlow, J. (1992). Social issues: An overview. In J. Bury, V. Morrison, & S. McLachlan (Eds.), *Working with women and AIDS: Medical, social, and counseling issues* (pp. 23-31). NY, NY: Tavistock/Routledge.

Boland, M. G., Allen, T. J., Long, G. I., & Tasker, M. (1988). Children with HIV infection: Collaborative responsibilities of the child welfare and medical communities. *Social Work*, 504-509.

Bowlby, J. (1980). *Attachment and loss: Loss, sadness, and depression* (Vol. III). New York: Basic Books.

Brazdziunas, D. M., Roizen, N. J. M., Kohrman, A. F., & Smith, D. K. (1994). Children of HIV-positive parents: Implications for intervention. *Psychosocial Rehabilitation Journal, 17* (4), 145-149.

Caldwell, M. Blake; Mascola, L., Smith, W., Thomas, P., Hsu, H., Maldonado, Y., Parrot, R., Byers, R., Oxtoby, M. (1992). Biologic, foster, and adoptive parents: Care givers of children exposed perinatally to human immunodefienciency virus in the United States. *Pediatrics, 90* (4), 603-607.

Carten, A. J., & Fennoy, I. (1997). African American families and HIV/AIDS: Caring for surviving children. *Child Welfare, LXXVI* (1),107-125.

Centers for Disease Control and Prevention, HIV/AIDS *Surveillance Report*. Midyear Edition, Vol. 9 (1).

Cohen, F. L., & Nehring, W. M. (1994). Foster care of HIV-positive children in the United States. *Public Health Reports, 109* (1), 60-67.

Commerford, M. C., Gular, E., Orr, D. A., Reznikoff, M, & O'Dowd, M. A. (1994). Coping and psychological distress in women with HIV/AIDS. *Journal of Community Psychology, 22* (3), 224-230.

Conners, M. (1996). Sex, drugs, and structural violence. In P. Farmer, M. Conners, & J. Simmons (Eds.), *Women, poverty, and AIDS: Sex, drugs and structural violence* (pp. 91-124). Monroe, Maine: Common Courage Press.

Corea, G. (1992). *The invisible epidemic*. New York: Harper Collins.

Dansky, S. F. (1997). *Nobody's children: Orphans of the HIV epidemic*. Binghamton, NY: Harrington Park Press.

Draimin, B. (1993). Adolescents in families with AIDS: Growing up with loss. In C. Levine (Ed.), *A death in the family: Orphans of the HIV/AIDS epidemic* (pp. 13-23). New York: United Hospital Fund.

Fair, C. C., Spencer, E. D., Wiener, L., & Riekert, K. (1995). Healthy children in families affected by AIDS: Epidemiological and psychosocial considerations. *Child and Adolescent Social Work Journal, 12* (3), 165-181.

Faithfull, J. (1997). HIV-positive and AIDS-infected women: Challenges and difficulties of mothering. *American Journal of Orthopsychiatry, 67* (1), 144-151.

Fanos, J., & Wiener, L. (1994). Tomorrow's survivors: Siblings of HIV-infected children. *Journal of Developmental and Behavioral Pediatrics, 15* (3), 43-48.

Farmer, P. (1996). Women, poverty, and AIDS. In P. Farmer, M. Conners, & J.

Simmons (Eds.), *Women, poverty, and AIDS: Sex, drugs and structural violenc* (pp. 3-38). Monroe, Maine: Common Courage Press.

Gardner, W., & Preator, W. (1996). Children of seropositive mothers in the U. S AIDS epidemic. *Journal of Social Issues, 52* (3), 177-195.

Gilbert, D. J. (1997). Catapulted development: The potential for rapid psychosoci: growth among women living with HIV/AIDS. Manuscript submitted for public: tion.

Gillman, R. (1991). From resistance to rewards: Social workers' experiences an attitudes toward AIDS. *Families in Society: The Journal of Contemporary Huma Services, 72,* 593-601.

Gillman, R. R., & Newman, B. S. (1996). Psychosocial concerns and strengths (women with HIV Infection: An empirical study. *Families in Society: The Journ of Contemporary Human Services, 77* (3), 131-141.

Groze, V., Haines-Simeon, M., & Barth, R. P. (1994). Barriers in permanency plar ning for medically fragile children: Drug affected children and HIV infecte children. *Child and Adolescent Social Work Journal, 11* (1), 63-85.

Hackl, K. L., Somlai, A. M., Kelly, J. A., Kalichman, S. C. (1997). Women livin with HIV/AIDS: The dual challenge of being patient and caregiver. *Health an Social Work, 22* (1), 53-62.

Juhasz, A. (1990). The contained threat: Women in mainstream AIDS documentar: *The Journal of Sex Research, 27* (1), 25-46.

Kaplan, M. S. (1995). Feminization of the AIDS epidemic. *Journal of Sociology an Social Welfare, 22* (2), 5-21.

Land, H. (1994). AIDS and women of color. *Families in Society, 75,* 355-361.

Lea, A. (1994). Women with HIV and the burden of caring. *Health Care for Wome International, 15* (6), 489-501.

Lesar, S., Gerber, M. M., & Semmel, M. I. (1995). *Exceptional Children, 62* (3' 224-237.

Lesar, S., & Maldonado, Y. A. (1996). *Children's Health Care, 25* (1), 19-35.

Lewis, S. Y., Haiken, H. J., & Hoyt, L. G. (1994). Living beyond the odds: . psychosocial perspective on long-term survivors of pediatric human immunodef ciency virus infection. *Developmental and Behavioral Pediatrics, 15,* (: S12-S17.

Lewis, M. (1995). The special case of the uninfected child in the HIV-affecte family: Normal developmental tasks and the child's concerns about illness an death. In S. Geballe, J. Gruendel, & W. Andiman (eds.), *Forgotten children of th AIDS epidemic* (pp. 50-63). New Haven, CT: Yale University Press.

Niebuhr, V., Hughes, J., & Pollard, R. (1994). Parents with human immunodefier ciency virus infection: Perceptions of their children's emotional needs. *Pediatric: 93* (3), 421-442.

Mellins, C. A., & Ehrhardt, A. A. (1994). Families affected by pediatric acquire immunodeficiency syndrome: Sources of stress and coping. *Developmental an Behavioral Pediatrics, 15* (3), S54-S60.

Michaels, D. & Levine, C. (1992). Estimates of the number of motherless yout orphaned by AIDS in the United States. *Journal of the American Medical Assoc ation, 268,* 3456-3461.

Miller, J., & Carlton, T. O. (1988). Children and AIDS: A need to rethink child welfare practices. *Social Work, 33* (6), 553-555.

Patton, C. (1994). *Last served? Gendering the HIV pandemic.* London: Taylor and Francis.

Risley-Curtiss, C., McMurtry, S. L., Loren, S., Gustavsson, N., Smith, E., & Faddis, R. (1997). Developing collaborative child welfare educational programs. *Public Welfare, 55* (2), 29-37.

Roberts, D. (1993). Child welfare services to drug-exposed and HIV-affected newborns and their families. In R. P. Barth, J. Pietrazk, and M. Ramler (Eds.), *Families living with drugs and HIV: Intervention and treatment strategies.* pp. 253-271, NY, NY: Guilford Press.

Sacks, V. (1996). Women and AIDS: An analysis of media misrepresentations. *Social Science and Medicine, 42* (1), 59-73.

Schable, B., Diaz, T., Chu, S. Y., Caldwell, M. B., Conti, L., Alston, O. M., Sorvillo, F., Checko, P. J., Hermann, P., Davidson, A. J., Boyd, D., Fann, S. A., Herr, M., Frederick, M. (1995). Who are the primary caretakers of children born to HIV-infected mothers? Results from a multistate surveillance report. *Pediatrics, 95,* 511-515.

Singer, M. (1992). AIDS and US ethnic minorities: The crisis and alternative anthropological responses. *Human Organization, 51* (1), 89-95.

Smith, D. K. & Moore, J. S. (1996). Epidemiology, manifestations, and treatment of HIV infection in women. In A. O'Leary and L. Sweet Jemmott (Eds.), pp. 1-24, *Women and AIDS: Coping and care.* NY, NY: Plenum Press.

Taylor-Brown, S. (1991). The impact of AIDS on foster care: A family-centered approach to services in the United States. *Child Welfare Vol LXX,* (2), 193-209.

Taylor-Brown, S. (1993). HIV-positive women: Finding a voice in the AIDS pandemic. In V. J. Lynch, G. A. Lloyd, & M. F. Fimbres (Eds.), *The Changing Face of AIDS* (pp. 123-147). Westport, CT: Auburn House.

Tiblier, K. B., Walker, G., & Rolland, J. S. (1989). Therapeutic issues when working with families of persons with AIDS. In E. D. Macklin (Ed.). *AIDS and families.* NY: Harrington Park Press.

Thompson, M. (1993). Drug-exposed infants and their families: A coordinated services approach. In R. P. Barth, J. Pietrazk, and M. Ramler (Eds.), *Families living with drugs and HIV: Intervention and treatment strategies* pp. 238-252, NY, NY: Guilford Press.

Wilton, T. (1997). *EnGendering AIDS: Deconstructing sex, text and epidemic.* Thousand Oaks, CA: Sage Publications.

Working Committee on HIV, Children, and Families. *Families in crisis: Report of the Working Committee on HIV, Children, and Families* (July 1997). NY, NY: Federation of Protestant Welfare Agencies, Inc.

Mothers with AIDS: Coping, Support, and Ability to Plan for Their Children

Sally Mason
Wynne Korr

SUMMARY. As the number of HIV-infected women increases, providers and policy makers are faced with an additional challenge–the number of children who will be affected by a parent's death from HIV. This paper reports the findings of an exploratory study of the relationship between coping of mothers with AIDS and the status of their plans for the future of their children. Nineteen women with an AIDS diagnosis and having regular contact with their children were interviewed. A chance health locus of control, the ability to cope with the death of others, availability of informal support, and a better health status were associated with more planning by mothers with AIDS. The findings suggest interventions for helping families plan and point to variables for future research. *[Article copies available for a fee from The Haworth Document Delivery Service: 1-800-342-9678. E-mail address: getinfo@haworthpressinc.com]*

KEYWORDS. HIV/AIDS, mothers, children, custody planning, permanency, coping, illness, support

---

Sally Mason, PhD, LCSW, is affiliated with the Institute for Juvenile Research, Department of Psychiatry, University of Illinois at Chicago, 907 South Wolcott (M/C 747), Chicago, IL 60612.

Wynne Korr, PhD, is affiliated with the School of Social Work, University of Pittsburgh, 2209 Cathedral of Learning, Pittsburgh, PA 15260.

[Haworth co-indexing entry note]: "Mothers with AIDS: Coping, Support, and Ability to Plan for Their Children." Mason, Sally, and Wynne Korr. Co-published simultaneously in *Journal of HIV/AIDS Prevention & Education for Adolescents & Children* (The Haworth Press, Inc.) Vol. 3, No. 1/2, 1999, pp. 119-141; and: *HIV Affected and Vulnerable Youth: Prevention Issues and Approaches* (ed: Susan Taylor-Brown and Alejandro Garcia) The Haworth Press, Inc., 1999, pp. 119-141. Single or multiple copies of this article are available for a fee from The Haworth Document Delivery Service [1-800-342-9678, 9:00 a.m. - 5:00 p.m. (EST). E-mail address: getinfo@haworthpressinc.com].

© 1999 by The Haworth Press, Inc. All rights reserved.

119

Although more than 80,000 children will be orphaned by AIDS by the year 2000 (Michaels & Levine, 1992), we know little about mothers with AIDS. Needs assessments indicate that a high percentage o women with HIV report having only one or no friends to help them cope with their illness or that of their children (Carr, 1990; LSC & Assoc., 1994). Isolation, stigma, and low income not only impair the family's functioning during the mother's illness, they may leave the parent with few options for placement of the children at her death This paper reports the findings of an exploratory study of how ability to cope with death, social support, health status, religiosity, socioeconomic status, and locus of control are associated with the status o mothers' with AIDS plans for their children's future.

BACKGROUND

HIV-Infected Women and Their Children

Women account for an increasing number and percentage of adult with AIDS (Ickovics & Rodin, 1992). In 1996, at least one out o every four people who tested HIV-positive was a woman (CDC 1996); some experts say the rate may be as high as one in three Women of color are especially impacted by HIV/AIDS–in 1996, 57% of women diagnosed with AIDS were African-American; 19% were Hispanic (CDC, 1996). Though the public still believes injected drug use is the main route of transmission for women, in 1996, heterosexual transmission accounted for a slightly higher percentage of cases in women than injected drug use (CDC, 1996). Most women with HIV are poor and living on public entitlements. A needs assessment in a large Midwestern city (Carr, 1990) found that the majority of women with AIDS were single with children. Most of these children are no infected, but they are affected by their mother's illness.

Best interest standards in child custody cases have historically emphasized stability, continuity, and predictability as essential to a child' healthy development (Hall et al., 1996). When a parent is living with HIV disease, however, the certainty and predictability of her life and her children's lives is threatened (Nagler et al., 1995). The parent' health may have ups and downs with each bout of illness presaging terminal illness or even death. As her health fluctuates, a mother may be in and out of the children's lives, depending on the care of relative or friends. Because of stigma and discrimination, the children may be uncertain about who to trust with the knowledge of the parent's HIV status or how to talk about it with someone (McKelvy, 1993). Relationships with relatives may be disturbed or even disrupted when the family learns that the mother and/or a sibling has HIV/AIDS (Hackl et al., 1997). Children also worry about the loss of their mother and their own future if their mother is no longer able to take care of them (McKelvy, 1993).

Custody Planning and HIV

The permanency or custody planning literature is surprisingly lacking regarding parents with a terminal illness. One group that does have some characteristics in common with HIV-infected mothers is elderly parents of adult children with disabilities, especially developmental. Elderly parents are in a position to plan for dependent children because of the parent's impending death or physical deterioration. Investigations into the propensity of these parents to plan indicated that most dealt with the decision by not deciding. Substitute care was difficult to discuss, especially as the options were perceived as ugly and painful. The topic was avoided. Parents had made no concrete plans or assumed that children would live with a sibling or other relatives (Heller & Factor, 1988; Smith & Tobin, 1989).

Studies of parents with HIV replicate this finding–HIV-infected mothers may not make plans (Gamble, 1993). Adolescents in HIV-affected families may be even less likely to have plans in place than younger children (Draiman et al., 1992). The emotional pain of having to plan for one's death is acknowledged as a barrier in the planning process (Draiman et al., 1992; Nagler et al., 1995). Often planning is also difficult because mothers cannot identify a future caregiver for their children (Hackl et al., 1997; LSC & Assoc., 1994; Mason, 1995). Yet mothers with AIDS have articulated their belief that planning is beneficial for their children (Mason, 1995). Children's uncertainty and stress may be reduced simply by the knowledge that there is a plan for them (Hudis, 1995). If mother dies, the children's adjustment can be facilitated by a smooth transition into a new home; a well-planned transition offers the continuity and stability that children need to grieve (Nagler et al., 1995; Siegel & Freund, 1994). Although the research in this area is still developing, there is preliminary evidence that affected adolescents who know there is a plan in place are at less

risk for a variety of behaviors, including HIV risk, than affected ado
lescents without a plan (Rotheram-Borus, 1996).

The term "permanency planning" implies both a process and ar
outcome. Planning is a process made up of several activities that leac
to the outcome of a permanent placement. The domains, especially a:
articulated by Heller and Factor (1988), appear to follow a progressior
from thinking about the options to formalizing arrangements legally
A modified version of Smith and Tobin's (1989) and Heller and Fac
tor's domains (1988) provided a framework for defining permanency
planning in this study. Based on the low socioeconomic status of mos
mothers with AIDS, financial arrangements were eliminated. The re
maining dimensions were:

1. Residential:
   a. what future living arrangements does the parent prefer and/o
      expect? (outcome);
   b. what is the status of those living arrangements? (process).
2. Legal:
   a. what legal arrangements does the parent prefer and/or expect'
      (outcome);
   b. what is the status of the legal arrangements? (process).

Coping and Stress–Gender and Socioeconomic Status

Planning for the care of one's children because of a terminal illnes:
is a major death preparatory behavior. Not all people with a termina
illness are able to engage in such behavior. What factors predict HIV
infected women's ability to plan for their surviving children? Thi:
study used a cognitive model of stress and coping to identify factor:
associated with planning and to develop research questions.

According to the cognitive model (Moos & Schaefer, 1993), a sense
of mastery and control enhances successful coping. In turn, each suc
cessful transaction with the environment further develops mastery anc
a sense of control. For low-income women, the opportunities for mas
tery and control are limited and many barriers to coping exist. Re
stricted opportunities and numerous stressors may generate creative
strategies. However, lack of success can start a process of erosion tha
makes a positive self-image and effective coping increasingly unat
tainable. Dill and Field (1982) applied a four-step cognitive model tc
explain coping efforts by low-income women. In this approach, coping

is considered as a transaction between person and environment (Dill & Field, 1982; Germain, 1981). Through a series of coping phases, the person and her environment carry out a transaction intended to reduce the stress. Personality, personal resources, and social support may mediate the reaction to stress by affecting cognitive appraisal of the stressor and choice of coping strategies.

Locus of Control–Illness, Gender and Socioeconomic Status

A key personality variable in studies of coping with chronic illnesses, such as AIDS, is control. The expectancy that one's behavior either is or is not directly related to one's outcomes is called locus of control. Locus of control is based in the individual's experience of the causal relationship between behavior and its consequences (Reid, 1984; Wallston & Wallston, 1981). Felton and Revenson (1984) acknowledged that controllability is a "critical property of stressors" and studied the relationship between coping strategies and controllability of illness (p. 344). They hypothesized that controllability would be associated with the use of strategies that deal directly with the stress or alleviated the emotional distress. Uncontrollability would require strategies that have to distort reality or at least temporarily compromise, the implication being that in uncontrollable situations, so-called "negative" coping strategies might be the most effective way to cope.

An internal locus of control has traditionally been considered the most beneficial to the individual. The individual with a strong belief that she can control her own destiny is likely to be more alert to those aspects of the environment which provide useful information and, then, take steps to improve her environment (Rotter, 1966). External control has often been linked with a profound sense of helplessness, hopelessness, depression, self-denigration, or alienation–the implication being that external control is bad. However, a growing number of researchers disagree. In some instances stress is reduced by accepting circumstances. The most effective adaptive response may be to cease trying to gain control or find those areas that one has control over and maximize them (Reid, 1984).

The theory that an external locus of control may be adaptive acknowledges the effect of the environment on reinforcement of expectancy (Wallston & Wallston, 1981). Both women and people with a low socioeconomic status experience lack of control over the environment and a lack of power based on their subordinate status. If the

environment is a reinforcer, then we can assume that effective adapta
tion for those groups might be toward externality. Travis (1988) con
tends that women's planning strategies–more contingent on the live
of others than men's–also contribute to externality.

People shift toward externality when living with a chronic illnes:
Relationships with health care providers and dependency on othe
due to incapacitation foster the development of externality. Howeve
there are also indications that those who already have a more externa
locus of control should find it easier to adjust to an environment tha
does not permit a high degree of personal control, i.e., chronic illnes:
In health research, generalized locus of control scales have been sup
planted by health specific scales. A health locus of control scale wa
designed to provide more sensitive prediction of the relationship be
tween internality and health behaviors (Wallston, Wallston, & Deve
lis, 1987). Studies offer evidence of the construct validity of the healt
locus of control scale and demonstrate the effectiveness of using
health-related measure over a more generalized scale (Wallston, Wal
ston, Kaplan & Maides, 1976; Wallston & Wallston, 1981; Wall et al
1989).

Coping with Death

Because AIDS is a terminal illness, coping with death must b
considered as a mediating variable. People with a terminal illness g
through a process described as "self-mourning" (Attig, 1989). Self
mourning has tasks not dissimilar to those of grief and is an activ
process. One of the tasks is "relearning of the world" (p. 367) an
reflects the notion of mastery and competence. In an attempt to predic
coping with death, Robbins (1991) built on Bugen's study (1980
using the concept of death competency. Death competence is based o
the construct of perceived self-efficacy and has been demonstrated t
be a better predictor of coping with death than anxiety (Robbins
1991).

Social Support and HIV

The provision of social support should mitigate stress and facilitat
coping. Unfortunately, the stigma of HIV almost guarantees the disrup
tion of relationships with family and friends. Women with HIV are jus

as likely to be abandoned as men yet women may also be providing care for a sick partner or child or an elderly parent. Asking someone for help means also disclosing that one is infected with HIV and, perhaps, even that a child is infected. Because she is a potential target of fear, anger, and blame, a mother may want to keep her HIV status a secret from family and friends in order to protect her family, thus closing out potential sources of emotional and concrete support (Hackl, 1997; Smeltzer & Whipple, 1991). Women with HIV, alone and ill, are increasingly unable to care for their families and have few resources for future care of their surviving children (LSC & Assoc., 1994).

HIV-infected women are also less likely than men to have networks of fellow sufferers to turn to for advice or information. Still a relatively small group and without the forms of community available to gay men, women with HIV have no reason to know one another (Semple, et al., 1993; Stuntzner-Gibson, 1991). Access to groups of other women with HIV infection or AIDS may be difficult because women are not tested early or diagnosed properly. Without diagnosis, women cannot access benefits and services associated with a diagnosis of AIDS. Women with HIV, often poor and/or substance abusing, may be suspicious of mental health and social services for fear that they will take away their children. Poor women are also more likely to lack knowledge of or access to resources. Transportation and childcare have been identified as significant barriers to health and mental health care for poor women and their children (McGrath, 1990; Belle, 1984).

Religiosity and Health Status

The research with elderly parents suggests two other variables that affect planning status: religiosity and health status (Smith & Tobin, 1989). Elderly parents, like parents with HIV/AIDS, are in a position to plan for dependent children because of the parent's impending death or physical deterioration. If the parents' health status was poor, they felt the urgency of making plans more acutely and were more likely to plan. Religiosity also contributed to planning through spiritual support and enhanced feelings of competence.

RESEARCH QUESTIONS

The following research questions were examined in the study:

1. What is the relationship between health locus of control and planning?

2. What is the relationship between social support and planning fc children?
3. What is the relationship between mother's socioeconomic statu and planning?
4. What is the relationship between coping with death and planning?
5. What is the relationship between religiosity and planning?
6. What is the relationship between mother's health status an planning?

METHODOLOGY

Sample

Selection criteria were: women, 21 years old or over, diagnose with AIDS, who had children under the age of 16. The children had t be either living with their mother or in substitute care such as foste care, relative care, or a group home. Mothers of children in substitut care had to have a plan for reunification, demonstrate an intention t follow that plan and/or have regular visits with the children. An AID! diagnosis using the expanded Centers for Disease Control (CDC AIDS Surveillance Case Definition (1993), rather than HIV infectior was chosen as a criteria for inclusion in the sample in order to increas homogeneity in health status. The revised AIDS definition include some severe manifestations of HIV found in women and injectioi drug users (e.g., invasive cervical cancer, pulmonary tuberculosis, an recurrent pneumonia) that had not been included previously. Socia service providers in hospitals and social service agencies in the Chica go area who served women with HIV were approached and asked fo their help in recruiting women who met the study criteria.

The desired sample size was twenty. There were two consideration in choosing the sample size. The first was the exploratory nature of th study. The study also included an in-depth interview about the moth ers' plans for their children. In order to conduct lengthy face-to-fac interviews, sample size had to be limited. The second consideratio: was lack of access to women with AIDS because of their chroni health problems and their understandable reluctance to disclose thei HIV status to a stranger.

The Interview

Participants were given a choice for the setting of the interview: at their home or at the service provider's facility. Sixteen interviews were held in the woman's place of residence; the other three were held (1) in a shelter where the woman was receiving temporary housing; (2) in a substance abuse treatment center where the woman was receiving inpatient care, and (3) in an office at the residential facility where the woman lived.

Instruments

Locus of Control

The Multi-Dimensional Health Locus of Control Scale, a health-specific scale, was utilized (Wallston, Wallston, & Devellis, 1987). The 18-item scale consists of three six-item subscales. Each subscale measures beliefs about a different source of control over health: internal, powerful other, and chance. The reported internal consistency reliability (Cronbach's alpha) ranged from .67 to .77. The scales have fairly good criterion validity, correlating with subjects' state of health. The scales also correlate with other measures of locus of control (Wallston, Wallston, & Devellis, 1987).

The three subscales of health locus of control were scored individually and then standardized. Based on her highest score, each woman was categorized as having an "internal," "chance," or "powerful other" locus of control.

Death Competence

Bugen's Coping with Death Scale was used to measure death competence (Bugen, 1980). The scale was originally used to measure changes in attitudes towards death and dying after participation in a death education seminar. Recently, it has been tested for validity and reliability as a measure of death competence or willingness to participate in death preparatory behaviors. Internal consistency reliability was .89 with a test-retest reliability estimate of .91 after eight weeks (Robbins, 1991). The scale has good construct validity, correlating highly with death-preparatory behaviors.

The total score of the Coping with Death Scale was used as one variable. Imbedded in the Coping with Death Scale are two subscales coping with one's own death and coping with the death of others.

Socioeconomic Status

Socioeconomic status is the position a person holds in society base on income, employment, and educational attainment. Closed-ende questions were used to obtain data on socioeconomic status. A socio economic status variable was constructed based on the woman' source of income before HIV infection (employed or on public entitle ments) and her years of education. Current source of income was no included in the variable because of the homogeneity of the responses

Social Support

Social support refers to the resources outside the individual (infor mal or formal) that provide physical and emotional assistance in dail living. Formal supports are services provided by social service agen cies and clinics. Informal supports are friends, neighbors, relatives Open-ended questions and probes were used to obtain informatioi from participants about informal supports. Utilization of formal sup ports was obtained with a closed-ended question.

The informal support variable was defined as the number of peopl the participants had told about their HIV status and the number o people available for concrete and emotional support for the mothei Formal support was defined as the number of social services utilizei over the past year.

Religiosity

Religiosity refers to the role that religion or spirituality played ii the women's lives. Intensity of religious/spiritual beliefs and extent o church involvement were obtained using closed-ended questions Open-ended questions were used to determine the impact of thei beliefs on coping with HIV. Religiosity was operationalized as thi woman's rating of her intensity of belief and her reported level o church participation.

Health Status

All of the participants had an AIDS diagnosis. Health status wa: conceptualized as health condition, including HIV and non-HIV re lated physical and mental health problems. The woman's report of her health was measured using open and closed ended questions. The mother's health status variable was constructed from the cumulative number of reported infections, whether or not she had been hospitalized for an HIV-related illness, and the woman's own rating of her health.

FINDINGS

Sample Characteristics

Nineteen women who met study criteria consented to participate. Nine were referred from a child welfare agency with specialized services for HIV-affected families; two from a residential facility; four were self-referred, and four came from HIV case management programs. The women ranged in age from 26 years to 43 years with a mean age of 34. Eight of the participants were African-American, seven were White, three Hispanic, and one was Native American/Jewish. Five had never been married, four were married or cohabiting with a male partner, eight were divorced or separated, and two were widowed, both by AIDS. The women's years of education ranged from 8 to 17. The mean and median number of years of education was 12 (see Table 1). Before diagnosis, employment was the source of income for the majority of the women. Fourteen of the participants reported Social Security Disability or Supplemental Security Income as their current source of income (see Table 1).

The 19 women were planning for a total of 47 children–23 girls and 24 boys. The children ranged in age from 1 year to 16 years with an average of 7.2 years. Most of the children (43) were 12 years old or younger. Seven mothers reported current Illinois Department of Children and Family Services (DCFS) involvement with at least one child. Twenty-eight children were living in the home with the mother; 19 were living in foster care or with some other caregiver. The mothers had from 1 to 5 children for whom they were planning with the average of 2.5 children per household. Two of the 47 children were HIV-infected.

Status of Plans for Their Children

Six planning activities, based on the domains suggested by the literature and on practice experience, were used to determine the plan-

TABLE 1. Characteristics of Mothers

Characteristic	Number
Age	
Range	26 - 43
Mean	34
Median	34
Race	
African/American	8
Caucasian	7
Hispanic	3
Other	1
Marital Status	
Single	5
Married/Cohabiting	4
Divorced/Separated	8
Widowed	2
Years of Education	
Range	8 - 17
Mean	12
Median	12
Previous Income	
Employment	13
AFDC	4
Prostitution/Dealing drugs	2
Present source of income	
SSI/SSDI	14
AFDC	3
Work Disability	1
None	1
Number of people living in household besides mother	
0 (lives alone)	6
1 other person	2
2	4
3	4
4	1
5	1
7	1

ning status: identified temporary caregiver in case of illness; identified potential caregiver in case of death; talked to caregiver about caring for children; received agreement from caregiver to care for children discussed details such as when they would take children or what the mother wanted for children; formalized plans with will, guardianship adoption, or standby-guardianship. The number of planning activities completed was used as the dependent variable in the remaining analy ses (see Table 2).

TABLE 2. Planning Activities Completed

No. of Activities Completed	Number of Women
6 activities	0
5	5
4	5
3	0
2	4
1	2
0 (none)	3

Relationship Between Variables and Planning Activities

The results of the statistical analysis are presented in Table 3. Given the small sample size, all variables (except health locus of control dimension) were dichotomized using a median split, e.g., high SES vs. low SES, more planning activities undertaken vs. less planning activities undertaken. Fisher's exact test was used to measure the association between planning status and each of the coping variables, except the dimensions of health locus of control. Fisher's exact test is recommended for 2 × 2 tables with small samples that may not meet the Chi-square criteria of a minimum count of 5 in each cell.

The greatest predictors of completion of more planning activities were a chance locus of control, an ability to cope with the death of others, a better health status, and the availability of informal positive support. Religiosity, date of positive test, socioeconomic status, and usage of formal support were not associated with planning.

The strongest association was between health locus of control and planning (p = 0.013). Women with a 'powerful other' (health professionals, family, friends) locus of control were less likely to have completed planning activities (see Table 4). Women with a 'chance' (luck, fortune, accident) locus of control were more likely to have completed planning activities. Women with an internal locus of control were equally likely to have been in the more or less planning categories.

Coping with the death of others was also significantly associated with planning (p = 0.023), while overall coping with death and coping with own death were not (p = 0.179 for both). The relationship between coping with the death of others and planning status was positive with higher levels of coping associated with more planning (see Table 5).

Health status and informal social support were both associated with

TABLE 3. Associations Between Coping Variables and Planning Status

Variable	p	
Informal Social Support	0.070	
Formal Social Support	0.170	
Religiosity	1.000	
Health status	0.070	
Positive test date[a]	0.656	
Coping with death	0.179	
of Self	0.179	
of Others	0.023	
Socioeconomic status	0.656	
Locus of control		
Internal/Chance/Powerful Other	0.0132	8.686[b]

[a] Dichotomized according to positive test date–1986-90 and 1991-93.
[b] Chi-square (Note–violates assumptions of chi-square).

TABLE 4. Health Locus of Control and Planning Status

Status	Internal	Chance	Powerful Other	TOTAL
Less planning	3	1	5	9
More planning	4	6	0	10
TOTAL	7	7	5	19

TABLE 5. Coping with Death of Others and Planning Status

	Low Coping	High Coping	TOTAL
Less planning	7	2	9
More planning	2	8	10
TOTAL	9	10	19

planning (p = 0.070). In the case of health status, better health was associated with more planning. The relationship between informal support and planning was positive–more informal support predicts more planning (p = 0.070). (See Tables 6 and 7.)

DISCUSSION

This discussion also draws on the findings from another part of the study. In a semi-structured interview, the mothers were asked about their plans for their children including: desired outcomes; the steps in planning; the advantages and disadvantages of planning; and the emotional legacy that the women wanted to leave with the children. This qualitative data informs our understanding of the findings on coping, support, and planning.

Chance Locus of Control

Chance played a role in at least one-third of the women's lives as evidenced by the health locus of control scores. The concept of chance

TABLE 6. Health Status and Planning Status

	Low Health	High Health	TOTAL
Less planning	6	3	9
More planning	2	8	10
Total	8	11	19

TABLE 7. Informal Support and Planning Status

	Low Support	High Support	TOTAL
Less planning	7	2	9
More planning	3	7	10
Total	10	9	19

or uncertainty was also evident in their descriptions of their illness an(
their approach to life. The potential of "here today, gone tomorrow'
was consonant with the literature on coping and illness. The quantit·
of life, if not the quality, is uncertain with HIV disease.

In that context, it is not surprising that the mothers wanted th·
opportunity to choose a caregiver for their children and could no
identify any disadvantages to planning. With planning, a mother coul(
reestablish her sense of control and affirm her competence as a mothei
Planning represented hope and certainty for her children's future
Planning could make one aspect of her world predictable. We woul(
expect a chance locus of control and more planning to be associated.

This finding, however, is contradictory to much of the traditiona
coping literature. That research would predict the strongest relation
ship between internal, not external or chance, locus of control an(
instrumental behaviors such as planning. This study's findings cal
into question the applicability of the traditional model to mothers witl
AIDS. Some of the recent work cited in the literature review on th·
adaptive function of an external locus of control seems more applica
ble. Since the women felt they had limited control over the length o
their lives, they looked for those aspects that were within their control
such as planning for their children. The women's coping may also b·
seen as "participatory" (Reid, 1984). They relinquished some contro
to a social worker or family member but were instrumental in seekin·
that help or promoting an alliance. Although the sample was small, th·
findings suggest that traditional coping models may not predict plan
ning behavior and support further development and testing of model·
that explain the intersection of women's coping, illness, and locus o
control.

Social Support

With HIV-infected mothers, the availability of positive informa
support may mean a larger pool of potential caregivers from which t(
select. People in the informal support network may also play a rol(
directly by encouraging the mother to make a plan or, indirectly, b)
freeing up time and energy so she can plan. Formal support was no
significantly associated with planning status perhaps because of th·
lack of variability in the sample: all of the women had formal suppor
through at least one social service agency.

Coping with the Death of Others

The relationship between coping with death and more planning was supported by the literature. In this study, the relationship was strongest with coping with others' deaths. Two women mentioned seeing other women with HIV get ill and die as triggers to planning. Perhaps, the ability to cope with anybody's death–whether your own or someone else's–is important for planning. However, this group of women may have found it easier to cope with another person's death or had more experience coping with another person's death than with their own.

Health Status

The researcher expected that poorer health would be related to more planning because women with declining health would feel the need more acutely to plan. The findings indicate the opposite. Perhaps women with better health have more energy to plan. Planning may also be easier to think about and, thus, easier to do when the need for the plan does not seem imminent. This finding may also be a function of the construction of the health status variable. The women's health ratings may have been more a measure of their health that day rather than an overall assessment of their HIV disease. The health status variable may also have been unreliable because of inconsistencies in the women's recall of the infections they had experienced.

Case Examples

Sandra had all of the characteristics associated with more planning–high health status, high informal support, high coping with others' death, and a 'chance' locus of control. She had completed four of the planning activities for both of her children–two girls who were 8 and 10 years old, the youngest also HIV-infected. Sandra had talked to an attorney about completing a stand-by guardianship and was waiting for the law to go into effect. About a year before the research interview, she had gone to court to get custody of her two daughters from their abusive father. She had given the children to their father years ago and was very pleased that she was able to provide for them again. She had told everybody in her life that she had HIV, including making public appearances. She identified several close friends that she could

count on. One of them was her next-door neighbor. She could no
think of a time when she had hoped to get help and had not received it
She had never been hospitalized, had never had any infections, an
rated her heath as excellent. Sandra spoke proudly of her recovery an
of the strength she received from the 12-steps. When asked wha
triggered her to take action in planning for her children, she said,

> The disease is so funny, you know, you could be here today an
> next week get sick and die and be healthy just like me. I mean
> have this fear that, I know I'm healthy now, but who know:
> what's gonna happen a week or two from now. One of thes
> bacterias that are already in my body could take over or I coul
> eat something that'll make me sick with bacteria.

Flora had all of the characteristics associated with less planning
low health status, low informal support, low coping with others' death
and 'powerful other' locus of control. Two of her children were in
kinship foster care, each with a different relative. The third child,
14-year-old boy, moved between her house and his father's home
few blocks away. She selected the foster care providers and the fathe
as the permanent caregiver but had only talked to one of the thre
about taking the children or about her HIV status. Her children did no
know of her HIV status either. She knew she needed to tell the care
givers and the children soon because she had just done a televisio
advertisement for a drug recovery program in which she identifie
herself as a person with AIDS.

Flora had three infections, had not been hospitalized, and rated he
health as fair. She said that her fiance and a volunteer helped her witl
concrete tasks such as transportation or shopping when she needed it
She had no one she counted on for emotional support. She said there
were "not too many people I can trust." She sobbed as she talke
about sitting alone in her apartment, feeling hurt and afraid, praying to
God to give her the "opportunity to show my kids how much I love
them." She talked at length about her difficulties with the child wel
fare system, trying to demonstrate to them that she was responsibl
enough to have her children again. Yet she expressed concerns abou
her ability to take care of the children full-time. She also had problem
with one of the relative foster parents. The paternal grandmother di
not trust her with her daughter and spoke poorly of her in front of th
child. The situation was made worse by the fact that Flora was relian

on public transportation to get to the suburb where they lived and rarely had the money to get out there.

Study Limitations

The small number of available subjects precluded random selection and limited data collection to those families in contact with a social service agency or health clinic. This contact, no matter how insignificant, may have been a variable affecting permanency planning. Isolated women, without access to health care or social services, were not represented in the study. The assistance of service providers in respondent identification may have biased the sample through selection of what each provider considered the "best" participants, although providers were asked to refer all women who met the study criteria. The small convenience sample in this study also precluded an in-depth study of race, ethnicity, or culture.

IMPLICATIONS AND CONCLUSION

The findings suggest some factors for consideration when providing custody planning services to HIV-infected mothers and their children. First, planning should be introduced early in the disease process while the parent's health is still good. Early planning allows for the time necessary to complete an emotional and complicated process while preventing crisis-based decisions. Building informal support may enhance the ability of a mother to plan for children, whether by increasing the network of potential caregivers or by introducing her to other mothers who are struggling with HIV. The support group is an intervention that has been used successfully throughout the epidemic. Groups may be particularly helpful with planning as they address two of the key variables in the study. Groups combine the development of informal support with the opportunity for women to see how other parents handle these issues, specifically coping with potential death.

The findings on locus of control, although only suggestive, indicate that practitioners and researchers should be wary of how we apply coping theories which do not take into account the stigma of HIV as well as the impact of race/ethnicity, gender, and socioeconomic status. The significance of a "chance" locus of control to many of the mothers reinforces the value of approaches which normalize the need to plan while acknowledging that many life events are beyond our control. Parents should pla not just because of HIV but because, in the mothers' words, "any of u could get hit by a bus tomorrow." When separated from the potential c death, planning is less threatening. Parents can take control of the proces rather than feeling controlled by their illness.

Future research should investigate other important variables in plan ning. Longitudinal studies of planning can help mental health profes sionals understand the changes in plans over time and the family dy namics during the process. We would also benefit from learning mor about the characteristics of women who plan and the strategies that the employ. For example, strong kinship networks and kin caregiving ar customary in African-American and Latino families (Chachkes & Jen nings, 1994; Martin & Martin, 1985; Stack, 1974). In these instances natural networks are already in place to support HIV-affected familie through a parent's illness or in caring for the children after a parent' death. Because informal caring has historically been a part of thos cultures, intervention by a professional or formal helping system ma be intrusive to the families' natural methods of caring and coping.

HIV disease also has different meanings in different cultures, carry ing more or less stigma. Family members may need education an counseling in order to come to terms with the parent's illness an continue to be supportive to the parent and the children (Chachkes & Jennings, 1994; Johnson-Moore & Phillips, 1994). Spanish-speakin parents and extended family members may want to plan but lac access to appropriate services (Chachkes & Jennings, 1994).

More research is essential to our understanding of the plannin process for HIV-affected families and the development of relevan programs and interventions. With planning, HIV-affected childre may be less vulnerable to a host of health and mental health problem whether their own risk for HIV or the long-term emotional conse quences of unresolved grief. Parents with HIV/AIDS can make th best decisions for their children, including transitions that suppor continuity and predictability.

REFERENCES

Attig, T. (1989). Coping with mortality: An essay on self-mourning. *Death Studies 13*, 361-370.

Belle, D. (1984). Inequality and mental health: Low income and minority women. I L.E. Walker (Ed.), *Women and mental health policy*, 135-150. Beverly Hills: Sage.

Bugen, L.A. (1980). Coping: Effects of death education. *Omega, 11,* 175-183.

Carr, A. (1990). *Summary of research report: The health care and social service needs of HIV-positive women and children in metropolitan Chicago.* Visiting Nurse Association of Chicago.

Centers for Disease Control and Prevention. (1992). 1993 Revised classification system for HIV infection and expanded surveillance case definition for AIDS among adolescents and adults. *Morbidity and Mortality Weekly Report, 41*(RR-17), 1-13.

Centers for Disease Control and Prevention. (1996). *HIV/AIDS Surveillance Report.* Public Health Service: Atlanta, GA.

Chachkes, E. & Jennings, R. (1994). Latino communities: Coping with death. In Dane, B.O. & Levine, C. (Eds.), *AIDS and the new orphans: Coping with death,* 77-100. Westport, CT: Auburn House.

Dill, D., & Field, E. (1982). The challenge of coping. In D. Belle (Ed.), *Lives in stress: Women and depression,* 179-196. Beverly Hills: Sage.

Draiman, B., Hudis, J., & Segura, J. (1992). *The mental health needs of well adolescents in families with AIDS.* New York: New York City Human resources Administration, Division of AIDS Services.

Felton, B.J., & Revenson, T.A. (1984). Coping with chronic illness: A study of illness controllability and the influence of coping strategies on psychological adjustment. *Journal of Consulting and Clinical Psychology, 52,* 343-353.

Gamble, I. (1993). *In whose care and custody.* New York: New York City Human Resources Administration, Division of AIDS services.

Germain, C. (1981). The ecological approach to people-environment transactions. *Social Casework, 62,* 323-331.

Hackl, K.L., Somlai, A.M., Kelly, J.A., & Kalichman, S.C. (1997). Women living with HIV/AIDS: The dual challenge of being a patient and caregiver. *Health & Social Work, 22,* 53-62.

Hall, A.S., Pulver, C.A. & Cooley, M.J. (1996). Psychology of best interest standard: Fifty state statutes and their theoretical antecedents. *The American Journal of Family Therapy, 24,* 171-180.

Heller, T., & Factor, A. (1988). Permanency planning among black and white family caregivers of older adults with mental retardation. *Mental Retardation, 26,* 203-208.

Hudis, J. (1995). Adolescents living in families with AIDS. In Geballe, S., Gruendel, J., & Andiman, W. (Eds.) *Forgotten children of the AIDS epidemic,* 83-94. New Haven, CT: Yale University.

Ickovics, J.R. & Rodin, J. (1992). Women and AIDS in the United States: Epidemiology, natural history, and mediating mechanisms. *Health Psychology, 11,* 1-16.

Johnson-Moore, P. & Phillips, L.J. Black American communities: Coping with death. In Dane, B.O. & Levine, C. (Eds.), *AIDS and the new orphans: Coping with death,* 101-120. Westport, CT: Auburn House.

LSC & Associates. (1994). *Report on the lives of Chicago women and children living with HIV infection.* Report submitted to Illinois Department of Children and Family Services to fulfill contract #176409013.

Martin, J. & Martin, E. (1985). *The helping tradition in the black family and commu-nity.* Silver Spring, MD: National Association of Social Workers, Inc.

McGrath, E., Keita, G.B., Strickland, B.R., & Russo, N.F. (Eds.) (1990). *Women and depression: Risk factors and treatment issues.* Washington, D.C.: American Psy-chological Association.

McKelvy, L. (1993). The Well Children in AIDS Families Project: A hospital-based program. In Levine, C. (Ed.), *A death in the family: Orphans of the HIV epidemic,* 104-109. New York: United Hospital Fund.

Michaels, D., & Levine, C. (1992). Estimates of the number of motherless youth orphaned by AIDS in the United States. *Journal of the American Medical Associ-ation, 268,* 3456-3461.

Moos, R.H., & Schaefer, J.A. (1993). Coping resources and processes: Current con-cepts and measures. In L. Goldberger & S. Breznitz (Eds.), *Handbook of stress: Theoretical and clinical aspects* (2nd ed.). New York: Free Press.

Nagler, S., Adnopoz, J., & Forsyth, B.W.S. (1995). Uncertainty, stigma, and secrecy: Psychological aspects of AIDS for children and adolescents. In Geballe, S., Gruendel, J., & Andiman, W. (Eds.) *Forgotten children of the AIDS epidemic,* 71-82. New Haven, CT: Yale University.

Reid, D.W. (1984). Participatory control and the chronic-illness adjustment process. In H.M. Lefcourt (Ed.), *Research with the locus of control construct (Vol. 3),* 361-389. London: Academic Press.

Robbins, R.A. (1991). Bugen's coping with death scale: Reliability and further val-idation. *Omega, 22,* 287-299.

Rotheram-Borus, M.J. (1996). Improving children's adjustment when the parent is living with AIDS. Paper presented at Role of Families in Preventing and Adapting to HIV/AIDS, Official Satellite Conference of the XI International Conference on AIDS, Office on AIDS, National Institute of Mental Health, NIH.

Rotter, J.B. (1966). Generalized expectancies for internal versus external control of reinforcement. *Psychological Monographs: General and Applied, 80,* 1-28.

Semple, S.J., Patterson, T.L., Temoshock, L.R., McCutchan, J.A., Straits-Troster, K.A., Chandler, J.L., & Grant, I. (1993). Identification of psychobiological stress-ors among HIV-positive women. *Women and Health, 20,* 15-36.

Siegel, K. & Freund, B. (1994). Parental loss and latency age children. In Dane, B.O. & Levine, C. (Eds.), *AIDS and the new orphans: Coping with death,* 43-58. West-port, CT: Auburn House.

Smeltzer, S.C., & Whipple, B. (1991). Women and HIV infection. *Image: Journal of Nursing Scholarship, 23,* 249-256.

Smith, G.C., & Tobin, S.S. (1989). Permanency planning among older parents of adults with lifelong disabilities. *Journal of Gerontological Social Work, 14,* 35-59.

Stack, C. (1974). *All our kin: Strategies for survival in a black community.* New York: Harper & Row.

Stuntzner-Gibson, D. (1991). Women and HIV disease: Am emerging social crisis. *Social Work, 36,* 22-28.

Travis, C.B. (1988). *Women and health psychology: Mental health issues.* Hillsdale, N.J.: Lawrence Erlbaum Associates.

Wall, R.E., Hinrichsen, G.A., & Pollack, S. (1989). Psychometric characteristics of the Multidimensional Health Locus of Control scales among psychiatric patients. *Journal of Clinical Psychology, 45,* 94-98.

Wallston, K.A., & Wallston, B.S. (1981). Health locus of control scales. In H.M. Lefcourt (Ed.), *Research with the locus of control construct (Vol. 1),* 189-243. London: Academic Press.

Wallston, K.A., Wallston, B.S., & DeVellis, R. (1987). Multidimensional health locus of control scales. In K. Corcoran, & J. Fischer (Eds.), *Measures for clinical practice: A sourcebook,* 239-241. New York: Free Press.

Wallston, B.S., Wallston, K.A., Kaplan, G.D., & Maides, S.A. (1976). Development and validation of the health locus of control (HLC) scale. *Journal of Consulting and Clinical Psychology, 44,* 580-585.

Index

© 1999 by The Haworth Press, Inc. All rights reserved.

T - #0577 - 101024 - C0 - 229/152/9 - PB - 9780789008251 - Gloss Lamination